FAT STUDIES

THE BASICS

Fat Studies: The Basics introduces the reading of fat bodies and the ways that Fat Studies, as a field, has responded to waves of ideas about fat people, their lives, and choices.

Part civil rights discourse and part academic discipline, Fat Studies is a dynamic project that involves contradiction and discussion. In order to understand this field, the book also explores its intersections with race, class, gender, sexuality, age, disability, ethnicity, migration and beyond. In addition to thinking through terminology and history, this book will aim to unpack three key myths which often guide Fat Studies, showing that:

1   fat is a meaningful site of oppression intersected with other forms of discrimination and hatred;
2   to be fat is not a choice (but also that a discussion of choice is itself problematic); and
3   fat cannot be unambiguously correlated with a lack of health.

Fat Studies: The Basics is a lively and accessible foundation for students of Gender Studies, Sociology, Psychology, and Media Studies, as well as anyone interested in learning more about this emergent field.

May Friedman is a Professor at Toronto Metropolitan University, Canada. Her research explores Fat Studies and unstable identities.

The Basics

The Basics is a highly successful series of accessible guidebooks which provide an overview of the fundamental principles of a subject area in a jargon-free and undaunting format.

Intended for students approaching a subject for the first time, the books both introduce the essentials of a subject and provide an ideal springboard for further study. With over 50 titles spanning subjects from artificial intelligence (AI) to women's studies, *The Basics* are an ideal starting point for students seeking to understand a subject area.

Each text comes with recommendations for further study and gradually introduces the complexities and nuances within a subject.

ANTHROPOLOGY OF REPRODUCTION
SALLIE HAN AND CECÍLIA TOMORI

SCIENCE COMMUNICATION
MASSIMIANO BUCCHI AND BRIAN TRENCH

PROJECTION DESIGN
DAVIN E. GADDY

ETHNOGRAPHY
SUSAN WARDELL

BAYESIAN STATISTICS
THOMAS J. FAULKENBERRY

FAT STUDIES
MAY FRIEDMAN

PROPAGANDA
NATHAN CRICK

For more information about this series, please visit: www.routledge.com/The-Basics/book-series/B

"This is an introduction to Fat Studies that is so much more than the basics. Friedman deftly weaves together the multiple histories and theories that are shaping Fat Studies today. The result is intersectional and accessible but never simple. It will be an invaluable touchstone for the field."

Francis Ray White, University of Westminster

"*Fat Studies: The Basics* brilliantly unpacks the complexities of fatness across social, cultural, and political facets of life. The book highlights the impact of fatness within healthcare and how media representation curates our perceptions of the body, revealing how dominant systems take up fatness and create inequities in all aspects of our lives. Each chapter evokes a thoughtful process to rethink the biases and assumptions that permeate our understanding of fatness, and encourages us to enter our everyday lives with a more nuanced understanding of inclusion, access, and body diversities."

Sonia Meerai, Assistant Professor, Laurentian University

"This accessible little primer dives into the biggest ideas emerging from Fat Studies today, debunking myths and exploring the rich history and realities of fat lives. A must-read for anyone interested in social justice and body politics!"

Carla Rice, Professor and Research Chair in Feminist Studies and Social Practice, University of Guelph

FAT STUDIES

THE BASICS

May Friedman

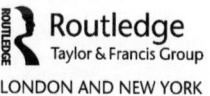

LONDON AND NEW YORK

Designed cover image: FlashMovie, Getty Images

First published 2025
by Routledge
4 Park Square, Milton Park, Abingdon, Oxon OX14 4RN

and by Routledge
605 Third Avenue, New York, NY 10158

Routledge is an imprint of the Taylor & Francis Group, an informa business

British Library Cataloguing-in-Publication Data
A catalogue record for this book is available from the British Library

ISBN: 978-1-032-88810-1 (hbk)
ISBN: 978-1-032-87941-3 (pbk)
ISBN: 978-1-003-53977-3 (ebk)

DOI: 10.4324/9781003539773

Typeset in Bembo
by Taylor & Francis Books

To all the Fat Studies students over the years who have blown my mind with your vulnerability and wisdom. This is for you.

CONTENTS

ACKNOWLEDGEMENTS

I swore I would never write another sole-authored book—too clunky, too many words to hold in my mind at once. The opportunity to write this book occurred unexpectedly after I taught my course *Fat Studies and Fat Activisms* at Toronto Metropolitan University in 2024. The cohort of students was so astonishing and that course stands out as one of the best teaching experiences I have ever had. If I had been approached at any other time I think I would have said no to writing a book about Fat Studies (a terrifying undertaking for so many reasons!) but the courage of those students wouldn't let me go—and here we are. First and foremost, my thanks goes to that group.

To my work family, especially JP—I wouldn't be standing without you and I owe you more than I can possibly convey. To my friend family, especially Marcia, Emma, Emily, Anna and Rachelle—you keep me going when it feels impossible. To my family, you are my reason for breathing. Sabrina and Danni— thank you for being our family, and Sab, thanks for being on so much of this journey with me and ahead of me. Dan, Noah, Molly, Izzy and Sasha—I will never stop being grateful for the lessons you teach me. I can't believe that this is my life.

INTRODUCTION

INTRODUCTION

As a species, we are characterized most of all by our variability. While all humans share the majority of our DNA in common, we come in a huge range of presentations: different skin tones, hair textures, facial features, heights and, of course, weights (National Human Genome Research Institute). While we are defined by our differences, not all of the ways in which we differ are treated equally. Some are treated as benign—for example, left-handedness. Others, such as gender identity or sexuality, are ascribed systems of meaning and political decision making.

Fatness is one form of human physical variation that is loaded with meaning. While fat people have always existed, and continue to exist in every known human society, associations with fat have varied across time and place. That said, fat people have been noteworthy for much of human history and are given particular attention in the present day.

This book will look at the lives of fat people, past and present, to try to understand how fatness is experienced and storied. This book will consider fat lives, and also the theories about them, which are now becoming grouped together into a discipline known as Fat Studies, an emergent field that considers body size as a site of discrimination and oppression and explores the variables of fat life.

FAT VS. FAT STUDIES: THINKING FATLY

While this book is officially about the study of fat—Fat Studies—it is impossible to think about fat theory without thinking about fat

DOI: 10.4324/9781003539773-1

life. This book will aim to debunk many of the key ideas that are commonly held about fat people—which is a central aim of Fat Studies scholarship—and also explore the specificity of particular fat lives. As a result, at points this book may seem like it's more about "Fat: The Basics" than about the particularities of fat scholarship, but at this stage, much of the theoretical work continues to be enmeshed with fat activism and the drive for fat liberation, so the overlaps will exist throughout the book, as they do in life.

Examining fat life is itself a theoretical undertaking that can truly re-program our way of thinking. While the focus of this book will be on unpacking fatness specifically, thinking about fat can also help us understand more about the world more broadly. For example, themes of citizenship, personal responsibility, health, religiosity, race and gender are all threaded through our understanding of fat lives and the rules, policies and laws that attempt to govern them.

This chapter is framed by the following questions:

- Why do we use the word "fat"?
- What are the histories of fat activism?
- What is "Fat Studies"?

WHAT DO WE MEAN BY "FAT"?

While "fat" is just a word to describe a way of being or a substance, the word is far from neutral. Instead, fat people have, historically and into the present, been viewed negatively. Fat folks are assumed to be lazy. Fat is associated with a lack of hygiene and self-care. Fat people may be seen as sexless or, in opposition, as oversexualized, especially with regard to fat women. Fat people are assumed to be ugly, with many popular representations of the fat love interest as the butt of a joke. Most of all, fat people are seen as gross—people who violate the social contract to be neat, tidy and contained. Much of our societal concern with fat people is rooted in this visceral "ick" that we've been taught to associate with fat people. We may even feel this disgust with our own fat bodies, or with people we otherwise love. The relationship between fat, shame and disgust is hard to unpack but is essential to an understanding of fat life and Fat Studies, because so much of the reaction to fatness is coming from this embodied ick.

Of course, while all of these associations are placed on fat people, they are simply untrue. Fat people come in the same range of embodiments and experiences as any other group—there are fat people who smell delightful and some who don't like to bathe. There are fat people with deep commitments to time management and others who struggle with procrastination. Ascribing any characteristics to a whole group of people is the essence of stereotype and should be viewed with great caution. Unfortunately, this caution is often ignored in thinking about fat people where the assumption that the stereotypes are rooted in reality is greatly taken for granted. (This is especially true in overwrought concerns about fat people's assumed poor health, something that will be taken up in greater detail in Chapter 4.)

This initial chapter will lay the groundwork for the rest of the book. We begin with issues of terminology, considering first and foremost the choice to centre the word "fat" and the complex messages which that word contains. This chapter will explore histories of the body and the ways that body policing is held in relation to colonialism and racism, laying a groundwork for the current state of fat stigma. The chapter will then move to a consideration of fat activism, including acknowledgment of formal and informal attempts to counter fat hatred and centre fat experiences. Particular attention will be paid to the ways that the seeds of fat reclamation originated with Black feminist thought. Finally, the chapter will examine the field of Fat Studies and consider how this academic approach to fat stigma and fat activism has come together in the last 15–20 years and how its approach may be fruitful in thinking through many different areas of privilege and oppression.

A NOTE OF CAUTION

It is tempting to dismiss all the "old" and "wrong" ideas about fat and replace them with new, enlightened ways of knowing about fatness. To replace one set of set beliefs with another, however, is contrary to the spirit of Fat Studies, which seeks, above all, to allow imperfection, improvisation and debate. There is no right way to feel about fat—your own or anyone else's. We live in societies that have a lot of opinions about fat people and it is therefore very difficult to feel neutral about fat lives and fat bodies.

Prioritize your own wellness and consider this book as an invitation to join a conversation, not to foreground a new "correct" way to think and live. Exposing the deeply held belief systems that may inform your personal and political relationship with fat can be uncomfortable, but can also be very exciting!

Fat Studies is still willing itself into being—with every year there are more publications, public events, activist encounters and private and public moments that are growing the project of Fat Studies, fat activism and public fat life more broadly. As a result, this is a dynamic and flowing movement. This book aims to begin to shut down stereotypical and dangerous perceptions of fat people and to allow for a range of possible alternatives to emerge. The book will help you understand both what Fat Studies is and what it has emerged in response to, but when the book is finished, Fat Studies, and the many different, intersected and complicated lives of fat people, will carry on, so consider this "The Basics—For Now", with room to participate in an ongoing and never-ending conversation.

While the unstable nature of Fat Studies can be frustrating, especially to folks who want to get a beginners' understanding of the field, it is also consistent with the political approach to fat life which craves a multiplicity of views and lived experiences. There are so very many ways to live and Fat Studies and fat activisms aim, at their best, to avoid proscriptive notions of a "right way". In this respect, it can be tempting to see Fat Studies as merely oppositional, rather than having an essential characteristic of its own. While this is a dynamic space, however, the overall commitment to love, beauty, discussion and debate, and the revelling in self-expression and joy, are definitional to the fat project and these are themes which will be explored in greater detail over the course of the book.

- As you read this book, it may be helpful to consider your own relationship to fat.
- What are your stories about fat people and fat bodies?
- How old were you when you learned about the concept of fatness? What people and systems taught you?
- What is your personal relationship to fat?

Fat is deeply societal and political, but it's also very personal. Our understanding of fashion, culture, health, society and beyond are all informed by how we feel about our own bodies and those of the people around us. If concepts in this book are new, consider why you may not have encountered them elsewhere. If they provoke feelings of distress or doubt, consider thinking through that discomfort and questioning where these feelings began.

WHY DO WE USE THE WORD "FAT"?

Words matter. They allow us to explain how we exist in the world, albeit imperfectly. They are a tool to describe our environments. Words can be tremendously empowering, but they can also do enormous harm. In the realm of thinking about people who are larger, the words we use are very important.

The choice to use the word "fat" is deliberate and has a long history. Because fat is often seen as a mean-spirited word, many euphemisms are often used in its place: curvy, fluffy, plus-size, ample, big-boned. While the desire to avoid hurting people's feelings—or contributing to our own humiliation—makes a lot of sense, ultimately the retreat to these alternate words says a lot about how much we have soaked the word fat with poison. We do not, for example, come up with complicated alternatives to calling someone double-jointed. We readily refer to people as tall—but might pause before using the word "short", especially to describe someone male-identified, knowing that there are social complications to living as a shorter man. Our fear of particular words gives them power.

At the same time that the word fat may feel weird or mean in our mouths, other words have gained currency. As we increasingly live in a world that is governed by science and health discourses, fatness has stopped describing a general range of possible bodies and has come to live at fixed points that are termed "overweight" and "obese". These terms draw from the Body Mass Index which suggests that BMI over 25 is overweight and over 30 is obese. (People with a BMI over 50 are considered, medically, "super morbidly obese".) While this book will delve into the problems with BMI more thoroughly in Chapter 4, its origins are far from pure. BMI was invented as a crude marker for describing human size, and its capacity as a diagnostic and organizational tool overlooks most sites of human diversity including gender, race, ethnicity, class and beyond. It's not by mistake that the person who invented the first tool that led to BMI, Adolphe Quetelet, was a famous eugenicist who sought to organize humans into many different categories for the purposes of understanding who was worthy and unworthy (Jacobs 2023; Strings 2023).

- Do you use the word fat to refer to yourself? Why or why not?
- Would you use that word to describe someone else?
- How does the word "fat" feel to you when you think about using it in everyday life?

BMI markers—those "o" words—suggest that there are fixed and reliable outcomes that occur at set points in the BMI scale, but this is not true—there is huge variability across all sizes in terms of health conditions, mobility, flexibility, etc. There are other problems: "overweight" automatically suggests that there is a fixed normal weight for all humans that, somehow, two-thirds of North Americans are "over" (Jacobs 2023). "Obese" has come to stand in for even more shaming characteristics than the word fat—obese people are automatically assumed to be lazy and reckless, on a one way trip toward death. Yet the third of North Americans who are obese come in a range of health manifestations, employment statuses and human experiences. These words aim to flatten fat experiences and suggest that there is a one-directional correlation between being bigger and being worse. (This, despite the fact of several large scale studies that found that the lowest mortality rate is for people in the "overweight" BMI category (Flegal 2021)).

Fat, by contrast, is a loose descriptor. What is fat in figure skating might be average or small in chef school. While it is essential to think about our different experiences across the fat continuum, and to acknowledge that the level of mistreatment and distrust that is aimed at people does grow with bigger sizes, ultimately the word "fat" seeks to let us describe ourselves and our own bodies. A fat body can be many different things—some of them delicious and others that we may continue to struggle with in the face of rampant fatphobia. Fat activists may revel in the body's unruliness, the ample dripping folds and bulges. But ultimately, fat is a word that is increasingly re-imagined:

> In fat studies, there is respect for the political project of reclaiming the word fat, both as the preferred neutral adjective (i.e., short/tall, young/old, fat/thin) and also as a preferred term of political identity. There is nothing negative or rude in the word fat unless someone makes the effort to put it there; using the word fat as a descriptor (not a discriminator) can help dispel prejudice. Seemingly well-meaning euphemisms like "heavy," "plump," "husky," and so forth put a falsely positive spin on a negative view of fatness.
>
> (Wann 2009, xii)

For many reasons, then, fat activism has leaned into the word fat and, perhaps unsurprisingly, Fat Studies has done the same. While there are euphemisms for other fields that are adjacent to Fat Studies—Critical Weight Studies, for example—many of these tip into fat shaming or pathologizing discourses and further, aim to seek legitimacy. It is uncomfortable to use the word fat, and it is disruptive to suggest that fat could be worthy of academic study. It is precisely the tension of this discomfort that Fat Studies wants to explore and expose. Doing so allows us to consider all sorts of rule systems that force us to be compliant and obedient and to question who they serve. If we can lose our shame about the word fat, about our own fat, what can we let go of next?

To read this book you don't need to already feel comfortable with the word fat, or even with the fact of fat. But hopefully this book will provoke you to begin to unpack when and how that word came to assume so much power and what would need to happen for it to become a neutral way of describing some bodies and experiences, or, perhaps even a site of pride.

Who gets to use which words? I often say to others: I get to call myself fat but I don't get to decide what you want to be called. Because words are so powerful, and because fat is still largely understood as an unkind word to apply to someone, caution still needs to be exercised in using it. It's a word that many of us have come to understand as beautiful, but nonetheless, describing others around you as "fat" without consent can still cause harm. That said: don't use "obese" and "overweight" instead! If you don't have a reason to describe someone's body, just don't. And if you do have a good reason, focus in on what you actually want to know: "What size shirt should I order you?" "Are you comfortable in that chair or would you prefer this one?" Fat people are very used to their fat being hypervisible in public space but also ignored for fear of embarrassment. Please acknowledge our size when it matters (when reaching for the right sized blood pressure cuff, for example)—and leave us alone otherwise.

HISTORIES OF THE BODY

There are many different ways that the body has been theorized over time. In Western philosophy, Enlightenment mind–body dualism suggests that body and mind are fundamentally separate. Other philosophies, notably those of Michel Foucault, note a greater congruency between body and mind, suggesting that the body, and its context, matter to how we understand our fundamental selves. No matter which approach we take, we cannot divorce ourselves from our bodies –they are what make us, *us*. Some of us many be deeply aligned with our bodies and feel them as a natural extension of ourselves, there to do our bidding. Others may feel quite disconnected from our bodies and their functions.

In the context of identity politics, bodies are deeply present. It is impossible, for example, to consider a politics of disability without considering the body and what are considered to be "normal" or normative functions. Likewise, theories and politics around queer and trans lives deeply implicate the body and what it does in specific places and times. This may have to do with the specifics of sexuality or genitalia, for example, but extends beyond these realms into other ways of being, dressing, presenting or existing in space. These ideas are also present when we think about race: while it is a crude explanation of racism to merely suggest that bodies of different colours experience public space and life differently, it is also a reality that is rooted in the specific corporeal experiences of embodiment.

Perhaps unsurprisingly, then, in the realm of fat, the body is also important, in both contemporary and historical settings. While fat bodies have always existed, the symbolism which has been applied to them has been variable. In many different societies over time, fatness has symbolized wealth and health. As such, fat was synonymous with desirability and an enviable life. At the same time, in many different traditions, "excess" (a variable and inconsistently marked size) was associated with greed, a lack of self-control and presumed laziness (Hill 2011). While the benchmarks of "right" size vary across place and time, there is still a sanction placed on bodies that are considered, by some measure, to be "too" large. This appears to be true across every place and time. Further, specific intersections change the model for ideal body type: in different eras, fat was related to fecundity and appreciated in female identified bodies; in other eras such as today in many Western cultures, fat is viewed as inconsistent with healthy fertility and policed accordingly.

> Fat is a "floating signifier": It's hard to figure out what the "right" size "should" be because it's not actually real. Ultimately, each body has its own relationship with weight and other characteristics and there is no universal correct size or shape (or race or hair texture or boob shape or running speed).

The fat body has often been associated with the grotesque (Bakhtin 1968). Abject theory, drawing from the work of Julia Kristeva (1982), considers the ways that the body's workings are seen as somehow disgusting and unseemly as opposed to the higher workings of the mind.

An over-emphasis on the body as dripping, leaking or otherwise behaving in uncontained ways is often held alongside bodies of size, but other "different" bodies have had similar critiques levied at them. For example, bodies that operate outside of usual expectations because of disability and illness are often seen as broken or deficient; especially when the bodies' inner workings are revealed, such as with –ostomies or limb stumps, revulsion may follow. Kathleen LeBesco signals the inclination toward disgust in her book *Revolting Bodies* (2003), suggesting that the very bodies that invite scorn can also be rebellious and steer us toward alternate futures. Perhaps this orientation toward reclamation and revolt is part of the deep connections between fat activism and Black feminist thought. Before Fat Studies was a field of study, scholars like Audre Lorde and bell hooks were considering the ways that disobedient flesh both frightened and rebelled against systems of power. Sabrina Strings' wonderful book *Fearing the Black Body: The Racial Origins of Fatphobia* (2019) considers the ways that fundamentally, a fear of fat stems from racist logics. The co-evolution of scientific thinking about race and size were dependent on one another and fundamentally shared a privileging of white, male, contained and disciplined flesh.

Fat bodies are often ignored—there are no clothes, seats don't fit, physical and public space seems to suggest fat people don't (or shouldn't) exist. At the same time, fat bodies are also hyper-present as examples of disruption and disturbance. For example, a staple in 18th- and 19th-century freak shows was the presentation of people who were of extremely large size. These bodies were viewed as remarkable but also as monstrous.

In the current moment the racial origins of fatphobia are all too present. In an era where explicit racism by health care providers, for example, is against codes of ethics, pointing out that someone is fat and demanding body management such as weight loss may be a new way to regulate specific (often racialized and Indigenous) bodies. If, as we will explore in the next chapters, weight loss is an impossible goal, then prescribing it as therapy is simply cruelty. This cruelty especially targets Black, Indigenous and other people of colour using age-old arguments grounded in white supremacy and colonialism: that only an effort-filled life is worthy and deserving. The irony that most wealth is achieved by generations of theft is erased here in favour of an analysis that talks about "hard work" while overlooking the labour of the hardest workers.

Many different texts take up the story of Sarah Baartman, a Khoikhoi woman who was "discovered" by white colonial settlers who subsequently put her on display around the world as an example of a remarkable and flawed body. The specific focus was on the size of the most sexual parts of Baartman's body, specifically her large bottom and genitalia. The fetishization and brutalization of this woman continued after her death when parts of her body continued to travel around the world for public display. For more information see Strings 2019.

The focus on individual success, numeric indicators and linear expectations of effort and achievement, are all deeply embedded in colonial frameworks. The notion of policing one's own body and divorcing it from its natural workings—not to mention its relationship with the environment and ecosystems beyond the body—is a terrible theft. Left to our own devices, we might consider the possibility that bodies grow dynamically and inconsistently, like the fruit on our trees. We might detect that in the animal world there is deep variability within the same species. Instead, we have entered the Barbie Factory where each of us should vary only slightly from the original idealized mold.

"Barbie" was originally designed by Ruth Handler as a doll named after her young daughter. The doll varied greatly from most dolls of the time which were meant to look like babies. Instead, Barbie emerged as a busty babe whose sexuality was only limited by her lack of genitalia. Early feminists remarked on the impossibility of Barbie's physique: were she formed at the size of an average person she would be incapable of standing or walking:

We know that if Barbie were real, she would have impossible physical dimensions. She would break in half if she bent over because her bust is too large to be supported by the size of her waist, not to mention her tiny, perpetually pointed feet. And she doesn't have enough fat on her body to menstruate. For this image to be the standard of beauty is problematic, because it sets an impossible and unhealthy ideal.

(McCoy 2023, para. 12)

Unfortunately, one of the insidious impacts of colonialism is the spread of logics, objects and markets. Diet culture, weight loss supplements, low calorie food and an insistence on a specific version of "health", create and proliferate a culture that suggests that individual responsibility is the only predictor of success; and likewise that any challenges come from individual failures.

Logics of the body have varied across geographies and time frames, and into the present day the self-help and responsibility focus continues to morph and shift. While the last decade has seen an uptick in the language of body positivity and self-care, both ensure that the onus is still on the individual to expend significant physical, financial and mental resources on ensuring that the self or the body is not only maintained, but also now, loved. The body at rest is an affront to capitalism and as a result, the fat body, which is stereotypically seen as the epitome of stillness, becomes the site of total scorn and rage.

FAT ACTIVISM

As can be seen above, for as long as there have been people, there have been fat people. And for as long as there have been fat people, there has been some form of fatphobia, even if the target size and scope of the scorn has varied across time and place. Importantly, however, while there is a lot of internalized shame and pain among fat folks, there has equally always been a spirit of resistance. It is impossible to understand fat life, then, without thinking through fat activism. Fat activism means a lot of different things and, the same way that fatphobia shape-shifts across spaces and eras, similarly, resistance to fat hatred has occurred in a range of forms.

Charlotte Cooper's book *Fat Activism: A Radical Social Movement* (2016) examines many different waves of fat activism, including "proxies" for fat activism that focus on fat adjacent ideas or fields. Importantly, Cooper locates civil rights organizations such as the National Association to Advance Fat Acceptance and the Fat Underground, but also focuses on "ambiguous fat activism", fat research, fat community and other less obvious sites of activist engagement. For many under-recognized and under-theorized peoples, simply existing in public space is a key site of resistance. Fat people are expected to change, or disappear, and the fact that so many have failed to do so is, in and of itself, activism.

Often, the canonical story about fat activism frames it as a social movement that arose alongside feminist organizing in the 1960s and 1970s and coalesced into formal organizational structures such as NAAFA and its more radical offshoot, the Fat Underground (FU). Some of the formal activism around fat oppression was informed intersectionally by feminist and especially queer engagement. Many sources point to the 1983 publication of the collection *Shadow on a Tightrope: Writings by Women on Fat Oppression* as a pivotal moment for fat organizing. Unfortunately, as Farrell details,

> this origin story also constitutes a serious problem. Even with the caveat that often precedes its telling ("this is only one of the stories") the frequency with which this origin story is repeated means it is becoming more entrenched, situating fat activism as a largely US, white, lesbian movement. Its repetition flattens fat, erasing complexity and contradiction, ignoring other voices, many of whom do not necessarily see fat as the crisis area, but rather as one crisis area out of many.
>
> (2020, 31)

The focus on this canonical story of fat activism creates an idealized view of activist practice that discounts the ways that many different forms of resistance have been lived by lots of people over time. The specific resistance that lives in organized protest, spectacle, writing and the engagement with public space is not always available to everyone, and doesn't encompass the wide range of practices that reflect resistance and resurgence. Fat Studies seeks to document the range of possible ways that fat people have resisted and sought fat joy in the face of fat hatred.

While the language of body positivity and self-love has come into ascendency in the last decade, there has always been resistance around the policing of the body. This is especially true for bodies that live in the intersections of multiple types of sanction and containment. For example, there has been overlap between disability activism and fat activism (and of course, there are many

people who are fat and disabled who advocate for both simultaneously). Suggesting a hierarchy of good or bad bodies works
against many people who are not fat or who are identified outside
of their fatness. By framing an analysis that welcomes a range of
bodies and abilities, and refusing the logic of "good" and "bad"
bodies, fat activism and disability activism align.

Civil rights organizing around race has been essential to fat
activism. In the modern era, many of the strongest voices speaking back against the privileging of smaller bodies were Black
women. Audre Lorde, for example, in her *Cancer Journals* (first
published 1980), responded to the pathologizing of her body as a
larger Black lesbian with a cancer diagnosis—it is impossible to
see Lorde's advocacy without exploring all of these identities and
struggles as interconnected. Strings (2019) points to the historic
demonization of Black bodies as the origin story for fatphobia—
but as fat Black hatred took root in colonial spaces, it was always
accompanied by resistance. Fat Black women, as Shaw writes,
"embody disobedience" (2006). Black author, activist, academic
and politician Dr. Jill Andrew brings in this framing in her
advocacy to end weight and size-based discrimination through
human rights frameworks. Andrew writes that,

> Fat bodies are framed as uncanny, excessive, and literally bursting out
> of bounds … Similar to the framing of Black bodies, fat bodies have
> been socially constructed as out of control, lacking self-determination,
> and are often painted as an unhealthy menace to health care.
>
> (2020, 223)

Like many other lessons learned from Black folks, especially
Black women, the origins of resistance are often whitened up
and divorced from their origins. Radical organizing around size,
race and ability becomes sanitized and repackaged as body
positivity or self-love and the political potential of these movements is reduced to an individual desire for a bubble bath or a
low cut shirt. While it is tempting to see this removal as inno-
cently misguided, it allows for a focus that continues the same
theme that is embedded in diet culture: a focus on changing the
self instead of changing the world.

Sonya Renee Taylor's groundbreaking work *The Body Is Not an Apology* explores the power of radical self-love. Taylor suggests that:

> Radical self-love is deeper, wider, and more expansive than anything we would call self-confidence or self-esteem. It is juicer than self-acceptance. Including the word radical offers us a self-love that is the root or origin of our relationship to ourselves ... Using the term radical elevates the reality that our society requires a drastic political, economic, and social reformation in the ways in which we deal with bodies and body difference.
>
> (2018, 6)

Taylor reminds us that we love ourselves in order to love one another and demand a better and more just world.

Sometimes, just being alive is a form of resistance. Being alive and enjoying that life is especially powerful for fat people who have been taught to apologize and shrink their lives at every turn. There is a specific form of activism that can be seen in fat gatherings, especially those that celebrate the body. Fat swims, fat beach days, fat clothing swaps are all ways that fat people gather unapologetically and both find joy and build community. While on the face of it these actions may seem minor, they have a huge impact on fat people especially for folks who are only recently coming into fat awareness.

Like all forms of activism, there isn't a singular, unitary pathway to being a fat activist. Indeed, the suggestion of a narrow way forward replicates the exact problems that fat activism seeks to eradicate. We should not believe that there is a single way to look or live. We want there to be variation and respect across difference. As a result, there needs to be respect for a range of different activist practices and comfort levels.

Recently, I taught a class in which I bemoaned the recent rise of weight control drugs such as Wegovy and Ozempic. As I looked around the room at my 50 students, however, I realized that it was almost a statistical certainty that people in the class were currently taking these medications. Without a doubt all people in the room, myself included, were navigating some sort of body management practices. To lead with the idea of a perfect way of being a fat activist is to reproduce the same narrow thinking we seek to rebut. Instead, we need to have a huge and expansive toolbox that makes room for all of our incredible skills and capacities but also our varying vulnerabilities and comfort levels. In addition, this toolkit needs to recognize that our proximity to risk—of derision, of medical mismanagement, of child welfare involvement, of legal enforcement—is not equal across all fat bodies.

FAT ACTIVISM AND THE ARTS

For many fat activists, multi-sensory and artistic approaches respond to some of the need for better fat representation. The movement is filled with dance, poetry, artwork, photography and other resplendent offerings. There are more avenues of fat activist art than could possibly be mentioned in this text box, but here are two to get you started:

Photographer and visual artist Shoog McDaniel captures fat bodies in a range of ways, including often in nature. McDaniel's work often brings together multiple fatties and celebrates the parts of fat aesthetics that are most often the most hated—showcasing cellulite, capturing fat bodies jiggling underwater and displaying ample rolls layered upon one another. This work is radical in its insistence on uncontained fat bodies—as opposed to the inclusion of "plus size" models who look largely like mainstream models just sized up a tad. The work is explicitly political and makes what is meant to be viewed as ugly, beautiful. In addition, much of McDaniel's visual art insists on the need to take up space and refuse to withdraw from the public gaze. More info can be found here: http://shoogmcdaniel.com/about.

Academic and artist Allyson Mitchell uses textile, visual art, video, photography and many other formats to celebrate fat life. Much of Mitchell's work is in creating "happenings"; for example, through now defunct fat activist collective Pretty Porky and Pissed Off, or the recent Kill Joy's Kastle. These events are meant to be provocative but also playful, and foreground fat, queer joy. Mitchell also uses craft, so often scorned as "women's" art, to explore the textures and layers of fat life. For more information go to: http://allysonmitchell.com.

FAT STUDIES AS AN ACADEMIC DISCIPLINE

As with other identity-based academic fields such as Women's Studies, Black Studies and Sexuality Studies, Fat Studies grew directly out of activism. While theorizing about fatness has occurred for many years, often in the context of Women's Studies or Gender Studies courses, the more formal entrenchment of Fat Studies as a field is more recent.

In 2009 two key collections were published. In England, *Fat Studies in the UK* was published by Raw Nerve books. Simultaneously, *The Fat Studies Reader*, edited by Esther Rothblum and Sandra Solovay, was published by New York University Press. While other books on fat life had been published in the years prior, the two anthologies represented a key moment in the bringing together of Fat Studies and the use of that title for the emergent field that explores size discrimination and weight acceptance. In 2012, the academic journal *Fat Studies: An Interdisciplinary Journal of Body Weight and Society* was launched with Rothblum as Editor in Chief. This further solidified the field and led to a greater degree of legitimacy for the discipline. In the inaugural issue Rothblum wrote that "Fat studies scholars ask why we oppress people who are fat and who benefits from that oppression. In that regard, fat studies is similar to academic disciplines that focus on race, ethnicity, gender, or age" (Rothblum 2012, 3)

As a field, Fat Studies draws from identity politics movements that foreground specific embodiments as both worthy of study and also often underrepresented or overlooked. Though fat organizing and resistance is as old as humanity, the shift toward discourses of health, and specifically the rise in fears around obesity since the beginning of the 21st century have contributed to greater analysis of fat bodies and, as a result, new manifestations of fat hatred. Simultaneously, racist discourses rooted in the need for self-regulation are well served by the fat witch hunt: fat hate is often poorly disguised racism. It is unsurprisingly, then, that Fat Studies began to emerge in response to these trends. While the field of Fat Studies still receives scorn from more conservative circles, it has gained traction and its existence is no longer new and surprising.

The academic study of fat is desperately important, especially since so much fat hatred is driven by scientific and expert driven discourses: all the arts based and joy filled approaches in the world can't speak back in the face of what is deemed to be scientific certainty. That said, academia is not an accessible space and the moving of fat resistance into the ivory tower has entrenched some degree of elitism into Fat Studies and has contributed to the side-lining of specific fat experiences. As an academic field, Fat Studies has continued the "official" retelling of fat resistance and as a result is not as wide ranging as a truly liberatory field needs to be. The introduction to the 2020 anthology *Thickening Fat: Fat Bodies, Intersectionality and Social Justice* names this concern:

> Normative expectations have a habit of creeping into critical studies. Even the progressive field of Fat Studies has sometimes failed to treat gender, sexuality, race, ethnicity, class, indigeneity, citizenship, age, geography and ability to full analysis. The normative subject of the field still tends to be a young(ish), white, cisgender woman, and typically one who is from the Global North. Fat activist spaces, too, tend to materialize as white, middle-class spaces. Like other fields and activisms invested in counter-hegemonic culture-building, Fat Studies and politics run the risk of erring on the side of sameness at the expense of difference.
>
> (Rinaldi et al. 2020, 2)

Collections such as *Thickening Fat* seek to rectify this imbalance, and indeed, the discussion about the need for greater diversity and intersectionality is present in a wide range of Fat Studies spaces. The field continues to grow and shift in response to its many contributors and, as a relatively young field, has room to evolve more nimbly than its older counterparts. While Fat Studies is far from perfect, many of its manifestations in classrooms and texts aim to respond to concerns about marginalization, and to foreground diversity.

FAT IN THE CLASSROOM

While thinking through fat liberation has been a part of courses for many years, especially in the context of Women- and Gender Studies classrooms, in the last decade, dedicated Fat Studies courses have begun to sprung up in a range of post-secondary institutions.

Many begin as special topics courses without a permanent course code. That said, Fat Studies courses have begun to be permanently on the list of electives (i.e. non required courses that aren't always offered) in a few places.

> Some of my motivation in writing this book comes from teaching an open elective at my university on the topic of Fat Studies and Fat Activisms. This course is offered through the School of Social Work and takes up many of the same themes which inform this book. I'm always struck by how overwhelmed and engaged students are in this course, how much they name wishing that they could think about themes and ideas from Fat Studies in other parts of their academic and non-academic lives. The course is, quite frankly, humbling: students of all sizes and crossing every other identity category, show up and confront deeply held beliefs and hold space for one another to find different answers. It has been the most rewarding teaching I have ever done.

Fat Studies courses are an easy target for critiques of identity-based and social justice oriented education. Right wing responses generally point to the field as self-indulgent and encouraging of obesity (the latter might be accurate!). Progressive critiques point, justifiably, to the ways that uncritical responses to fat and body acceptance can maintain tropes of whiteness and self-discipline without actually providing structural critiques. Teaching Fat Studies can be exhausting in the face of all this criticism! That said, Fat Studies in the classroom makes a huge contribution. Students not only learn about the specificities of fat hatred and fat activism, but also are taught to cultivate scepticism about widely held beliefs that span many different parts of society. Fat Studies allows for an analysis of the interplay of policy and people as well as the many different ways that populations can be regulated, often through what seem to be our own "innocent" choices. As a result, the application of the skills gained in Fat Studies courses can allow students to become critical thinkers in ways that may extend to a range of other settings.

The political, of course, is always personal. I am astonished by how often students have commented about wishing that their mothers could learn about Fat Studies, in order to both change their relationships with one another, but also to heal mothers' own painful relationships to their own bodies. Fat Studies students learn to be critical and to question their own body management practices (all the things we all do, no matter how woke, to regulate our bodies in public space). This systems-level understanding, however, can result in tears and revelations, connections and breakthroughs. The class comes together as a community and every week there has been a feeling that we are uncovering something revolutionary.

While teaching Fat Studies is inspiring, there is also validity to the concerns about Fat Studies as a field. The most valid critique is that it is completely counterintuitive to teach about how we need to move away from striving for personal perfection within a colonial academic setting that makes students work for a grade. It's not a perfect field and these are not perfect classes. In sitting with such tender content, we may hurt one another, we may be more vulnerable than we can afford (instructors included!). That said, there is a lot of magic accomplished in these spaces.

FUTURE DIRECTIONS

As a relatively young field Fat Studies has only begun to scratch the surface of thinking through the body in space. Drawing from prior theorization of the body has allowed for a range of robust scholarship but there are so many fat populations and fat experiences that have not yet entered into formal scholarship and so many different bodies that are still under-represented or excluded. As with many identity based fields, Fat Studies can sometimes be overly populated by bodies that are the most normative: smaller, whiter, and overall less threatening to academic systems. It remains to be seen whether these bodies and these scholarships will blast open the fences of academia for more and more exceptionalities to enter, or whether they will close the gate behind them. In truth, it will likely be some combination of both. Future work in Fat Studies can learn from some of the pitfalls of, for example, second wave feminism, in order to create as expansive a tent of knowledge and learning as possible. There are so many possibilities and opportunities ahead!

Who are Fat Studies scholars? Because there is no formal academic department of Fat Studies anywhere in the world as of this writing, Fat Studies scholars are housed in a wide range of disciplines including Gender Studies, Sexuality Studies, Cultural Studies, Sociology, Social Work, and beyond. More and more emerging scholars are using Fat Studies as a theoretical and methodological framework for their work, so the field continues to grow and spread into many different academic spaces.

WHAT NEXT

At this point you've learned about why we might use the word fat, how bodies have been framed over space and time, and how fat activism has morphed into Fat Studies both formally and informally. Yet our understanding of Fat Studies is incomplete without a bigger understanding of the many different facets of weight stigma and fatphobia. In order to understand Fat Studies as a legitimate field, fat people must be understood as a distinct population with unique and important challenges and strengths. This is tricky, because of course fat life, like any other identity grouping, is varied and inconsistent. That said, moving along now we'll consider some of the costs of fatness and the ways that living while fat, though enormously variable, can nonetheless be seen as a meaningful site of identity worthy of discussion and response.

FURTHER READING

Cooper, Charlotte. *Fat Activism: A Radical Social Movement*. HammerOn Press, 2016.

Farrell, Amy Erdman. "Thickening Fat and the Problem of Historiography." *Thickening Fat: Fat Bodies, Intersectionality and Social Justice*, edited by May Friedman, Carla Rice and Jen Rinaldi, Routledge, 2020, pp. 29–39.

Meleo-Erwin, Zoe. "Queering the Linkages and Divergences: The Relationship Between Fatness and Disability and the Hope for a Livable World." *Queering Fat Embodiment*, edited by Cat Pausé, Jackie Wykes, and Samantha Murray, Routledge, 2014, pp. 97–114.

Strings, Sabrina. *Fearing the Black Body: The Racial Origins of Fat Phobia*. New York University Press, 2019.

WORKS CITED

Andrew, Jill. "Introduction." *Body Stories: In and Out and With and Through Fat*, edited by Jill Andrew and May Friedman, Demeter Press, 2020, pp. 13–19.

Bakhtin, Mikhail. *Rabelais and his World*. 1968. Indiana University Press, 1984.

Farrell, Amy Erdman. "Thickening Fat and the Problem of Historiography." *Thickening Fat: Fat Bodies, Intersectionality and Social Justice*, edited by May Friedman, Carla Rice and Jen Rinaldi, Routledge, 2020, pp. 29–39.

Flegal, Katherine M. "The Obesity Wars and the Education of a Researcher: A Personal Account." *Progress in Cardiovascular Diseases*, vol. 67, 2021, pp. 75–79.

Friedman, May, and Carla Rice and Jen Rinaldi, editors. *Thickening Fat: Fat Bodies, Intersectionality and Social Justice*, Routledge, 2020.

Hill, Susan E. *Eating to Excess: The Meaning of Gluttony and the Fat Body in the Ancient World*, Praeger, 2011.

Jacobs, Alexander E. "How Body Mass Index Compromises Care of Patients with Disabilities." *AMA Journal of Ethics*, vol. 25, no. 7, 2023, pp. 545–549.

Kaloski Naylor, Ann, and Corinna G. Tomrley, editors. *Fat Studies in the UK*, Raw Nerve Books, 2009.

Kristeva, Julia. "Approaching Abjection." *Powers of Horror*, Columbia University Press, 1982, pp. 2–6.

LeBesco, Kathleen. *Revolting Bodies? The Struggle to Redefine Fat Identity*, University of Massachusetts Press, 2003.

Lorde, Audre. "The Cancer Journals." *Disability Journals*, edited by G. Thomas Couser and Susannah B. Mintz, Macmillan Reference USA, 2019, pp. 110–114.

McCoy, Heath. "For Better and For Worse: Feminist Scholars Weigh In on Barbie's Legacy." *UCalgary News*, https://ucalgary.ca/news/better-and-worse-feminist-scholars-weigh-barbies-legacy, 2023.

McDaniel, Shoog. "Shoog McDaniel." http://shoogmcdaniel.com/about.

Mitchell, Allyson. http://allysonmitchell.com.

National Human Genome Research Institute. "Genetics vs. Genomics Fact Sheet." https://www.genome.gov/about-genomics/fact-sheets/Genetics-vs-Genomics.

Rinaldi, Jen, and Carla Rice and May Friedman. "Introduction." *Thickening Fat: Fat Bodies, Intersectionality and Social Justice*, edited by May Friedman, Carla Rice and Jen Rinaldi, Routledge, 2020, pp. 1–11.

Rothblum, Esther D. "Why a Journal on Fat Studies?" *Fat Studies: An Interdisciplinary Journal of Weight and Society*, vol. 1, no. 1, 2012, 3–5.

Schoenfielder, Lisa, and Barb Wieser, editors. *Shadow on a Tightrope: Writings by Women on Fat Oppression*, Aunt Lute Books, 1983.

Shaw, Andrea E. *The Embodiment of Disobedience: Fat Black Women's Unruly Political Bodies*, Lexington Books, 2006.

Strings, Sabrina. *Fearing the Black Body: The Racial Origins of Fat Phobia*, New York University Press, 2019.

Strings, Sabrina. "How the Use of BMI Fetishizes White Embodiment and Racializes Fat Phobia." *AMA Journal of Ethics*, vol. 25, no. 7, 2023, pp. 535–539.

Taylor, Sonya Renee. *The Body Is Not an Apology: The Power of Radical Self-Love*, Berrett-Koehler Publishers, 2018.

Wann, Marilyn. "Foreword: Fat Studies: An Invitation to Revolution." *The Fat Studies Reader*, edited by Esther Rothblum and Sondra Solovay, New York University Press, 2009, pp. ix–xx.

HOW FAT HURTS

INTRODUCTION

In the first chapter we explored issues of language and the different histories of the fat body and fat activism that bring us to the present day. There are critiques of fat activist practices from both conservative and progressive points of view. For many people, fat activism is seen as a huge indulgence—the most ridiculous example of equity and diversity initiatives gone wild. Why, detractors argue, should we worry about fat people when they are responsible for their own discomfort? Arguing from the perspective of social justice, there are concerns, sometimes valid, that centring fatness takes away from more "important" concerns such as racism. At the heart of these concerns, however, is a perspective that suggests that fat people don't truly suffer in ways that are similar to other sites of oppression. Drawing from Fat Studies scholarship, this chapter seeks to explain some of the impacts of living in a fat body and the ways that the structural oppression of fat folks—the systems that go beyond interpersonal insults—is embedded in day to day life, and from birth to death.

This chapter is framed by the following questions:

- What are the social consequences of living in a fat body?
- How do different intersections impact fat lives?
- How do different life stages change the experiences of fat life?

This chapter begins by explaining the ways that fat is a significant and measurable site of oppression. Exploring the consequences of

DOI: 10.4324/9781003539773-2

fat stigma from cradle to grave, the chapter will aim to consider many of the different ways that fat hatred and the exclusion of fat life occur. The chapter will take an intersectional focus, considering the ways that fat oppression is similar to, different from, and works with other identities and embodiments, themes that will be taken up more completely in Chapter 6.

FAT STIGMA: HOW DO FAT PEOPLE EXPERIENCE THE WORLD?

Fat people are the butt of the joke and even in politically correct settings are permitted to be the punchline. Fat stigma is so deeply embedded that sometimes a fat person needs only to appear for people to sneer or laugh. In common with many other sites of oppression, however, fat hatred is not merely the same as rudeness and can't be fixed by people being nicer. Rather, fatphobia is replicated and amplified in social structures that impact every area of people's lives. Living in a fat hating world teaches us that to be fat is bad and that we must be ashamed if we are fat and that we must avoid fat at all costs if this is not yet our reality. Fat is also an additive identity— the other social locations in a person's life intersect and interlock with fat.

Fat people experience the world as *emotionally hostile*. To be fat, while common, is to transgress the social contract. There is judgment and shame in every interaction. All food choices are observed and policed, from eating in public to consulting with a nutritionist for food related health concerns. "Health trolling", the phenomenon of bystanders heckling because they are "just concerned about your health" is on the rise. Beginning in childhood, parents may feel pressure to monitor children's bodies, physical activity, size and shape, in the name of both health and aesthetics.

Fat people experience the world as *physically uncomfortable*. Public spaces are not designed with fat bodies in mind, even though many people are fat. Public transportation, school seating and medical equipment not only pinch people's bodies—they convey the ways that bigger bodies are fundamentally wrong and that they should be excluded from public space. Fat people's needs are viewed as irrelevant to planning decisions. Owen terms this "spatial discrimination", the ways that the orientation of literal space works against fat folks (2012). They suggest that the arrangement of physical space ensures that fat people experience non-stop micro-aggressions that serve to remind people not only to stay home, but ideally, not to exist. Owen writes:

> From the moment a fat person awakes in the morning, s/he is reminded of living fatly in a thin-centric world. Shower stalls in which we have to stand sideways (baths are rarely an option); towels that won't fasten around our waists or chests; disproportionately expensive or ill-fitting jewelry, belts, shoes, and clothing; narrow doorways, hallways, aisles and bathrooms; too-tiny and/or molded plastic seats in buses and on subway trains; narrow, flimsy, or armed office, lawn, theater, airplane, restaurant, and dining room seating; weight limits on exercise equipment; hospital gowns, blood pressure cuffs, MRIs, life jackets, seatbelts, and other health or safety devices that simply don't fit: all are constant reminders that fat persons don't fit, that our most basic needs, desires, and safety therefore matter less.
>
> (2012, 294)

Fat activist academic T. J. Stewart puts the following disclaimer on his course outlines to make transparent the many ways that campus life is forbidding to bigger students:

> Fat Students & Students of Size: The reality is that many campus buildings and structures are either out of date and/or they have furniture or classroom structures that are not friendly or conducive for fat people or people of size. I always do my best to mitigate these issues but may not always be successful. At any time if you find yourself experiencing discomfort (physical or otherwise) particularly related to body-size as a result of fatphobic, anti-fat, or sizeist structures please let me know immediately. I will work with you on a solution or accommodations including finding suitable furniture, requesting a classroom change, or another alternative— so that you can have a better learning environment.

This statement led to a bigger research project by Stewart and others that sought to document the interrelated limitations of campuses for fat students (Stewart 2018).

Fat people experience *internalized fatphobia*. The extent to which "fat" is equated with "bad" is deeply engrained. While infants do not know to scorn their delicious rolls, by age five fatter children experience bullying and thinner children know to view fat young people as problematic or intrinsically flawed. Furthermore, it is nearly impossible to be fat without seeking to eliminate fat—the vast majority of fat people (and thin people) are engaged in some type of body management practice (diet or exercise or surgery or some combination). It is hard to love a body you are trying to erase. The deep shame many fat people experience is caused by fatphobia, but it also allows fatphobic beliefs to be maintained because, so often, folks are too embarrassed and humiliated to ask for their fat bodies to be treated with dignity and affection. Ironically, pervasive stigma and hostility contribute to stress, which can cause a host of health concerns, concerns for which fat people, of course, are blamed.

WHAT DO WE CALL WHAT FAT PEOPLE EXPERIENCE?

You may have noticed that there is a range of different terms that are applied to the oppressive experiences faced by fat folks. Many of these terms are used interchangeably in this book, but while the terms have common threads, there are specific differences between them.

Sometimes the discrimination against larger bodies is termed *size-ism*, reflecting the hierarchy in which particular sizes are viewed as more powerful and advantageous than others. Similarly, *weight stigma* explores the specific personal and institutional impacts of living in a larger body; so do *anti-fat* and *anti-fat bias*. These terms are meaningful in terms of engaging with systems and frameworks that draw on rights discourses and require specific mapping of experiences in order to convey discrimination. That said, these terms do not always acknowledge the breadth of experiences of both fat people and people who have any kind of relationship with fat (used to be fat, loving people who are fat, secretly hating your boss that is fat, questioning why you are so very worried about getting fat).

Fatphobia is a commonly used term, and what is beneficial about this term is that it acknowledges the extent to which the *fear* of fat may impact people of all sizes. In a world that is profoundly disrespectful and judgmental of fat people, avoiding fat becomes a society-wide concern. In common with other oppressive systems that use the language of "phobia" (homophobia and transphobia for example), the term reflects the deep disgust and fear of specific bodies and practices which characterize much of the common discourse around fat people and fatness generally.

I think about my grade school kids. We live in an urban centre where diversity is celebrated and, while there is obviously much unchecked racism, homophobia and transphobia and ableism in the classroom, at least the talk is "talked" about many human differences. The classroom is, however, oddly silent on the topic of fat, apart from the odd fat joke made by a child which doesn't get corrected. I realize that these sweet kids mostly celebrate their differences, do not fear coming out as queer or trans, proudly acknowledge their neurodivergence. I feel that if students knew they were going to grow up to be fat, however, they wouldn't have the same reaction. It's impossible to know, but given the ways they have encountered fat (obesity prevention in the health unit, fat villains in all their novels, lectures about fruit) this possible future stands apart from many others as a unique site of fear and revulsion. How does this affect all the kids in the class? What about the ones that are already larger than their peers?

Are you afraid of fat? Sometimes in public talks or classes I get challenged about whether fatphobia is in fact all around us. I will ask people of all sizes: "How would you feel if you gained 100 lbs from wherever you are now?" It turns out that, with very few exceptions, most people are deeply uncomfortable with the thought of a body that is substantially larger than present, no matter what size they currently are. Furthermore, if I amend the question and ask how folks would feel if they were 20–30 lbs lighter, most people admit that this would be welcome, even if they have already embraced fat activism as part of their lives. Consider asking yourself both questions and then reflect on what your response may reveal about your beliefs. If your first concern is about your health, perhaps reflect on where that belief was learned as well.

Sometimes we use the language of *fat hatred*. Given the over-whelming prevalence of language of "obesity epidemic", and the extent to which fat people have been blamed for moral disorder, impacts on public safety, and burdening the health care system, among so many other ills, it doesn't seem hyperbolic to suggest that "hatred" is the right word.

More recently, some scholars in Fat Studies have used the term *fatmisia*:

> Fatmisia ... is prejudice plus power; anyone of any weight or body type can have/exhibit size-based prejudice, but in North America and across the globe, thin people have the institutional power, therefore fatmisia is a systematized discrimination or antagonism directed against fat bodies/people based on the belief that thinness is superior.
>
> (Simmons University Library 2024)

Fatmisia links the hatred of fat people and fear of fat to larger institutional structures such as capitalism and patriarchy. As such, this term reflects the pervasiveness of anti-fatness and the ways it is deeply embedded in every possible aspect of human life. This embeddedness is explored further below as we examine the impacts of fatness across the lifespan.

All of these terms are useful and all help describe the life experiences of fat people and of all people in a fat hating society. There is specific impact from using particular words and most Fat Studies scholars use many of these different words throughout their writing.

MEASURING THE IMPACTS OF FAT LIFE

It's a hard world for anyone in a body bigger than what is accepted as "normal". These impacts start young and influence every stage of life as well as a range of different contexts. For example, before we are born, the fetal environment may be scrutinized for "obe-sogenic" influences, with the uterus we grow in already being viewed with suspicion. Concern about size and perceived health implications are offered throughout pregnancy, not only in the context of health care but also often by concerned bystanders see-mingly trained in eyeballing a perfect bump. Once we emerge, the fact that the pre-birth environment matters is conveniently erased

and we are immediately entered into a weight conscious matrix—
that the first "facts" that are offered about a new human are most
often sex designation and weight speaks volumes about our values
as a society and our passion for fixed systems of description and
measurement. As tiny infants we are expected to gain weight and
there is concern if we fail to do so, for perhaps the only time in
our lives. By the time we are toddlers, living outside of the bell
curve of the pediatric growth charts is suspicious and alarming,
despite the fact that these charts are not only organized by sex at
birth but also based on samples that are not at all representative of
human diversity (Sandler 2021).

Body self-consciousness begins very early in life. Children as young
as five express discomfort with bigger bodies and are aware of avoiding specific foods to attempt to change shape (Tatangelo et al. 2016).
Research asking young children to pick playmates from a range of
non-normative physicalities routinely finds that they pick fatter children last (Kornilaki 2014). Perhaps unsurprisingly, then, bullying of
fat children is overwhelming, conspicuous, and largely unaddressed
(Weinstock and Krehbiel 2009; Wei and DiSanto 2011). Despite a
climate that is increasingly attentive (at least theoretically) to mental
health concerns and bullying, fatness remains an easy target. The
relationship between fat and shame means that adults are reluctant to
acknowledge that fat kids are hypervisible, so uncomfortable social
interactions can be overlooked or underestimated. Unfortunately,
adults are not exempt from fatphobic views so they may also feel less
warmly toward fatter kids and/or make judgments of their parents. As
with all other areas of stigma, living within an oppressive system has
impacts on school performance, mental health and self-esteem. Fat
kids may be too self-conscious to participate in sports teams or
other sites of joyful movement (Flores Aguilar et al. 2020), ironically leading to "confirmation" that fatter people do not want to
move. Fat kids are singled out for diet and exercise advice more
than their peers—effectively all eyes are on fat kids, but, in contrast
to other identities, there is no pride or alliance to provide support.
Fat kids are thus both horribly overexposed to scrutiny and
simultaneously ignored.

By puberty the message that fat is always terrible and wrong has
become obvious, just in time for many kids who were smaller to
plump up in anticipation of coming body changes. These impacts

can be especially debilitating to trans or non-binary kids for whom puberty can be particularly overwhelming. Puberty can be, even for cisgender kids, a time where the body feels out of control, and the impact of added weight can cause emotional upheaval. Many young teens engage in body changing practices, including dieting or other food restriction or punitive exercising (Tanner 2023). The fearmongering about the "obesity epidemic" (explored further in Chapter 4) also ensures that medical practitioners are echoing the message of increased weight as both a body failure and also a failure of will. While health is the suggested goal of these messages, medical interventions into weight management in younger people have resulted in a much greater incidence of eating disorders. Registered dietician and author of *Unapologetic Eating*, Alissa Rumsey states that

> A child is 242 times more likely to have an eating disorder than they are to have type 2 diabetes. Yet the vast majority of our public health education is spent warning parents (and kids) about "childhood obesity". Why? Fatphobia, not health. If you took a sample of 100,000 children, only 12 would have type 2 diabetes … but 2,900 would meet the criteria for an eating disorder. By 9 years old, 50% of girls have dieted or restricted their food intake in some way.
>
> (Rumsey 2021)

If the majority of our health messages warn parents about "childhood obesity", we should be questioning what is happening. This messaging has led to a generation of dieters and is a sign that dieting is not really about health: in so many ways, diets actually make us unhealthy: physically, mentally and emotionally. Further, yo-yo dieting and other dramatic interventions can have lifelong impacts on metabolism, ironically harming overall physical health while also having impacts on mood and emotional wellness.

Strong4Life is a public health campaign put out by the state of Georgia. In 2011 the campaign featured billboards with photographs of fat young people with phrases such as "Warning: It's hard to be a little girl when you're not" and "My fat may be funny to you but it's killing me." Notably, many of the young people in the photos were kids of colour. In response, fat activists led by Marilyn Wann began the "I Stand Against Weight Bullying" campaign which sought to buy billboards and replicate the style of the images but to offer fat affirming phrases such as "I STAND against harming fat children. Hate ≠ health." The counter-campaign was itself somewhat controversial, tending initially to focus on white women's images and affiliating itself with Health At Every Size (in some respects, a problematic movement, to be discussed in the coming chapters). Nonetheless, this grass roots response was a meaningful moment in the history of both fat hatred and fat activism.

By adolescence young people are very aware of the hierarchy of acceptable bodies. Pride movements around sexuality and gender identity may build community and enhance well being; identity based activism around race and ethnicity place joy alongside experiences of racism and exclusion. For fat people, however, there may be no pride, no joy, and often, at younger ages, little access to activism or community. Fat adolescents are often excluded from dating and relationships (though assumptions of oversexualization may lead to fat young adults, especially those who are identified as female, being sexually harassed). Teachers may knowingly or unknowingly penalize fat students, falling into assumptions of laziness (Dian and Triventi 2021). Fat students may be less likely to be admitted to post-secondary education or offered scholarships.

By adulthood the penalties for fatness have become evident and extend throughout all aspects of life. Fat people are less likely to be hired and are overlooked for promotion (Flint et al. 2016). Fat people, who have often been doubted since childhood, may also lack the confidence to ask for what they need, in work and elsewhere in life. The saturation of shame in fat life can make it very hard to lead with confidence, especially when fat coincides with other experiences of marginalization. While this is not true for every single fat person, even people who are, for example, very confident in dating situations may still experience fat shame at doctors' offices.

Speaking of doctors' offices: they are not designed with fat people in mind, emotionally or physically. Doctors have been trained to be scrupulous about letting people know they're fat (as though fat people do not have access to mirrors?) and that fat is dangerous and deadly. As a result, fat people recount that virtually every doctor's visit for any reason is met with the suggestion of weight loss (Borisova and Stockelova 2024). Beyond the suggestion to lose weight, many fat people are met with explicit hostility in medical settings, some of which may verge on malpractice. Fat people with uteruses and/or breasts, for example, are offered Pap smears and mammograms less frequently than thinner people (Wee et al. 2000), resulting in less prevention for cancers. Accurate equipment (bigger blood pressure cuffs, longer needles, adequately sized MRI and CAT scanners) may not be available or offered, resulting in a lower quality of care, all of which is seen solely as the fault of the fat person.

In later life fat may be protective: for people over 55 "both overweight and obesity confer a significant decreased risk of mortality" (quoted in Bacon and Aphramor 2011, 2). Despite this, the onslaught of fat shaming and blaming discourses never ends. It is often acknowledged that thinness requires money—for healthy food, for gym memberships, for the leisure time required to engage in body maintenance—but fatness may also simply lead to poverty because of the more limited educational options, career possibilities and lack of confidence that fat people may experience. As a result, fat people are poorer, which makes retirement harder to achieve and may contribute to the many poorer health outcomes of low income. As all people grow older, physical health may become more complicated. For fat people, this inevitable shift is attributed to their fatness, so instead of just living in an older body, they are continuously treated as though they are in defective bodies.

Even at the end of life fat bodies continue to lack respect. Bigger coffins are more expensive and may be difficult to source. Not all crematoria have the capacity to care for supersized bodies. Our death systems, like those throughout our lives, are designed with specific bodies in mind, but these specificities do not acknowledge the range of embodiments that actually exist.

Where do we learn that fat is bad? Virtually every representation of a larger person in popular culture suggests that, at best, fat characters are lovable but messy (Winnie the Pooh) and at worst, disgusting and hateful (Dudley Dursley). Fat characters exist only to set up a redemption arc (Fat Monica on the sitcom *Friends*) or as the punch-line to a joke about an unattractive blind date. Fat Americans are shown as so damaged that they must look outside the country for love (in the context of *90-Day Fiancé*, insulting both fat and foreign experiences all at once!). Fat people are, by definition, miserable (*This Is Us*), unwell (*My Mad, Fat Diary*) and stupid (Homer Simpson). These ideas will be taken up in greater detail in Chapter 5.

Trying to find a fat character who is unremarkable, whose character traits are not predetermined by their size, is virtually impossible outside of explicitly fat activist media. Fat forward pop culture is amazing—shows such as *Shrill* or books such as *The Accidental Pinup* series—but such offerings are often preaching to the choir and are drowned out by the deluge of fatphobic offerings everywhere else. We make this media because of our biases but we also learn those biases from this media, thus ensuring that the negative associations with fat are maintained.

FAT AT THE INTERSECTIONS

The general trajectory for fat life is deeply challenging. While the challenges are all around us, the specifics of how fat people experience the world are informed by many other contexts and experiences. The specific messaging around fat is amplified in regard to particular identities and connections. While these themes will be taken up in more detail in Chapter 6, it is impossible to acknowledge the impacts of fat hatred without considering how it connects with other forms of oppression.

It's important to note that *all* fat bodies live intersectionally—no one is fat and nothing else. Identity analyses can be somewhat crude tools for understanding human experiences but specific identities can result in different structural experiences. Looking at a few of these experiences can remind us of the tremendous variability of fat life and also the alchemy of fatphobia as it mixes with other injustices.

In the realm of gender, fat life can be quite different for people who are male or female identified, and different again for folks who live outside of the binary. Fat women are hypersexualized or invisibilized from sexual expectations—either seen as insatiable or unlovable. The aesthetics of size are especially punishing to fat girls and women who are expected to disappear. Weight is deeply important, but so is shape—fat women must be cellulite and stretchmark free, with all curves being smooth and elevated. While standards have shifted in popular culture toward desire for thicker thighs and larger bums, overall there is still a very narrow realm of acceptability for women's body shape (Fikkan and Rothblum 2012).

Men's bodies may escape some of the punishment that is placed on women's bodies, though as the conversation increasingly highlights health instead of appearance (even though it is *all* about appearance), all people are expected to self-regulate at all times. That said, there is a wider range of normal for male-identified bodies. With that in mind, however, men may also be desexualized by flesh seen as excessive. Non-athletic men are seen as weak or effeminate, failing at the task of manliness by allowing rolls that may resemble more stereotypically feminine flesh.

While an androgynous aesthetic is increasingly seen as desirable, interestingly, this look is also framed around thinness. Most of the gender neutral clothing available for purchase is made in a narrow size range, and the popular culture version of non-binary life is often associated with a slim, flat body. Furthermore, the specifics of fat placement can gender bodies (though in very inconsistent ways—fat rolls may make a body more or less feminine or masculine depending on context and community opinions). For trans and non-binary folks the body may feel even more fraught, and controlling appearance and public reading of the body can be overwhelming (White 2014). Adding the chaos of fat to the mix can contribute to distress internally, but also to bullying and violence externally.

Across all intersections, fat can sometimes be easy to hate and mock. We live in a toxic and difficult world with a lot of hateful messages about difference, so arguably we have all taken on some degree of internalized racism, sexism, etc. If we have learned that it is impolite to express these views we may allow them to emerge in the context of fat hatred, which is still largely permissible, as a proxy for other forms of hatred. In other words, middle schoolers may bully the fat trans kid because they are fat, but also as a means of expressing their (unacceptable) transphobia. This can make it very hard to name oppressive behaviours because they are occurring in the in-between of different identity markers.

Even as we talk about microaggressions and aim to figure out how to hold space for kindness, so much of our experience of hatred—across all identities—occurs in the blurry middle ground of how we feel in the world. The world is filled with unbelongings—in fact there are almost as many ways to be a wrong person as there are people! We are constantly facing scrutiny and judgment and we may not always know why. We may also not know why we judge others: is the vague feeling of being grossed out that we get due to someone's size or the way they chew their food? Are we thrown off by a mismatch between ours and someone else's neurodivergences or is something more insidious at play? Only deep reflection can help us unpack the variety of poisons we've ingested. In the realm of fatphobia and especially where it bumps into other identities—as it does with virtually everyone—the hidden nature of fat shame and blame can make it even harder to untangle what is going on in any given interaction. As a result, fat folks may swallow a particularly large dose of unpleasantness, unwilling to call out racism because it is cloaked in fat shame, turning on themselves and their gender presentation because it's also related to their fat flesh. In the felt state, this in betweenness can be truly devastating.

Fat Studies theorizes connections between fat and disability. Authors have asked whether fat can be understood as a disability and, by the same token, the emphasis on fat as natural variation resists (some of) the language of disability. Nonetheless, when disability and fat co-occur, the language and treatment of fat people can be uniquely toxic. Fat people with mobility differences can be assumed to be the cause of their own difference; fat people with mental health differences are more easily understood as lazy or "crazy". While the over-valorization of people with disabilities is a real problem, the lack of any generosity toward fat bodies may result in the opposite effect: fat people with disabilities who are unworthy of anything other than scorn.

There are specific and insidious components to fat hatred toward Black, Indigenous and other people of colour. As explored briefly in Chapter 1, much of the contemporary face of fatphobia was birthed by colonization. The focus on weights and measures, the necessity for self-governance, the reification of a specific view of normalcy—these are all colonial structures. The overwhelming abuse and degradation of Indigenous people and communities included focusing on bodies as wrong, and on mocking and erasing traditional food and body practices. Into the present, one of the ways that Indigenous populations continue to be policed is in the over concern about diabetes. There is much funded research about obesity prevention in Indigenous populations in Canada, for example (Robinson 2020), but much less attention paid to how to support reparations for the overwhelming and unending impacts of colonization.

For Black communities, there is a similar fixation on health conditions such as heart disease, hypertension and diabetes—all conditions that are correlated with stressors caused by racism—but little support in maintaining livable lives (Roberts 2010). Fatphobia toward communities of colour is often a new face of racism that allows for the scrutiny of and vigilance toward folks of colour with a new judgmental frame: laziness due to fat replaces judgment due to colour. It is not by accident that some of the most offensive racist beliefs are similar to the stereotypes about fat people. Stoll writes that, "When it comes to race, fatphobia, which has always been intimately connected with the historical development of whiteness in the United States, is often used as a way to mask overt racism in the name of 'health'". (2019, 9) These judgments have deadly consequences: while there is an attempt to address explicit racism in healthcare, fatphobia allows for shaming and judgment of people of colour to continue; bigger Black kids may face even more punitive and shaming interactions in school settings; and, as Mollow displays, police violence against bigger Black bodies is not only occurring, but may then be storied as the fault of the victims themselves as a result of being Black and fat (2017).

This analysis isn't meant to offer a hierarchy of oppressions where, if you eat at the oppression buffet and your plate is more full you are therefore more pathetic. Rather, by exploring the specificity of some combinations of fat possibilities, we can consider the widest range of experiences and remember that fat phobia is a shapeshifter: it can be executed in innumerable different ways and exploits both personal and structural vulnerabilities.

WHERE DO WE GO FROM HERE?

It would be impossible to effectively list the many different consequences of fat life in contemporary societies. This chapter is not meant to be a definitive account of fat oppression but rather to note that fat hatred is worthy of our attention. In the quest for justice, fatphobia creates enough terrible consequences that it requires a commitment to its dismantling, a deep awareness of, and response to, the overwhelming scope of fat shame and hatred.

Alongside the many challenges to fat life it is deeply important to recognize the existence of fat pride, fat community, fat art, fat joy! Fat activist spaces reclaim fatness; many fat people revel in their ample bodies and do not see them as sites of misery and harm. This chapter seeks to articulate some of the difficulties fat people face, but no fat life is singular—we experience hate but also love; experience pain, but also joy. The reclamation of the word fat is partially an attempt to wrestle both the words and experiences of fat life from a narrative that is only about suffering. While it is important that this book—and the project of Fat Studies more broadly—acknowledges the many strands of fatphobia, it is equally important that these experiences are never viewed in isolation.

As previously discussed, Fat Studies and fat activism receive critiques from both progressive and conservative sources. The general consensus is that to think about fat is a self-indulgence, that fat hatred isn't really that bad and that to combat fat oppression steals resources from issues that really matter. Hopefully this chapter has begun to flesh out the many ways that fatphobia and fat hatred matter, the impacts across people's lives and interlocking with many other oppressions. Of course, the major reason why the many impacts of fat hatred do not persuade people from both right and left is because of one of the abiding myths about fat that Fat Studies seeks to debunk: that fat, unlike other identities and conditions, is fundamentally a choice and that, if fat folks don't want to be treated poorly, they should choose not to be fat. It is this myth, then, that we turn to in Chapter 3.

FURTHER READING

Owens, Lesleigh. "Living Fat in a Thin-Centric World: Effects of Spatial Discrimination on Fat Bodies and Selves." *Feminism & Psychology*, vol. 22, no. 3, 2012, pp. 290–306.

Stoll, Laurie C. "Fat Is a Social Justice Issue, too." *Humanity & Society*, vol. 43, no. 4, 2019, pp. 421–441.

Wann, Marilyn. "Foreword: Fat Studies: An Invitation to Revolution." *The Fat Studies Reader*, edited by Esther Rothblum and Sondra Solovay, New York University Press, 2009, pp. ix–xx.

WORKS CITED

Bacon, Lindo, and Lucy Aphramor. "Weight Science: Evaluating the Evidence for a Paradigm Shift." *Nutrition Journal*, vol. 10, no. 9, 2011, pp. 1–13.

Borisova, Varvara and Tereza Stockelova. "This Doctor Knows Shit about You, but the First Thing He Says Is 'You Need to Lose Some Weight': Anti-Fat Bias and the Contradictory Effects of Fat Medicalization in Czech Healthcare." *Fat Studies: An Interdisciplinary Journal of Weight and Society*, 2024, pp. 1–19. DOI: doi:10.1080/21604851.2024.2381920.

Dian, Mona, and Moris Triventi. "The Weight of School Grades: Evidence of Biased Teachers' Evaluations against Overweight Students in Germany." *PLoS ONE*, vol. 16, no. 2, 2021.

Fikkan, Janna L., and Esther D. Rothblum. "Is Fat a Feminist Issue? Exploring the Gendered Nature of Weight Bias." *Sex Roles*, vol. 66, 2012, pp. 575–592.

Flint, Stuart W., Martin Čadek, Sonia C. Codreanu, Vanja Ivić, Colene Zomer, and Amalia Gomoiu. "Obesity Discrimination in the Recruitment Process: 'You're Not Hired!'" *Frontiers in Psychology*, vol. 7, 2016.

Flores Aguilar, G., M. Prat Grau, C. Ventura Vall-Llovera, and X. Ríos Sisó. "'I Was Always Made Fun of for Being Fat': First-Hand Accounts of Bullying in Children's Football." *Physical Education and Sport Pedagogy*, vol. 26, no. 6, 2020, pp. 549–561.

Kornilaki, Ekaterina N. "Obesity Bias in Preschool Children." *Hellenic Journal of Psychology*, vol. 11, 2014, pp. 26–46.

Mollow, Anna. "Unvictimizable: Toward a Fat Black Disability Studies." *African American Review*, vol. 50, no. 2, 2017, pp. 105–121.

Owens, Lesleigh. "Living Fat in a Thin-Centric World: Effects of Spatial Discrimination on Fat Bodies and Selves." *Feminism & Psychology*, vol. 22, no. 3, 2012, pp. 290–306.

Roberts, Dorothy. "The Social Immorality of Health in the Gene Age: Race, Disability and Inequality." *Against Health: How Health Became the New Morality*, edited by Jonathan M. Metzl and Anna Kirkland, NYU Press, 2010, pp. 61–71.

Robinson, Margaret, "The Big Colonial Bones of Indigenous North America's 'Obesity Epidemic.'" *Thickening Fat: Fat Bodies, Intersectionality and Social Justice*, edited by May Friedman, Carla Rice, and Jen Rinaldi, Routledge, 2020, pp. 29–39.

Rumsey, Alissa. [@alissarumseyRD]. *Instagram*, February 17, 2021a, https://www.instagram.com/p/CLZR4K_noeg/?igshid=14ek0g5zmbxwj&img_index=2.

Rumsey, Alissa. *Unapologetic Eating: Make Peace with Food & Transform Your Life*, Victory Belt Publishing, 2021b.

Sanders, Rachel. "The Color of Fat: Racializing Obesity, Recuperating Whiteness, and Reproducing Injustice." *Politics, Groups, and Identities*, vol. 7, no. 2, 2019, pp. 287–304.

Sandler, Austin. "The Legacy of a Standard of Normality in Child Nutrition Research." *SSM – Population Health*, vol. 15, 2021, pp. 1–9.

Simmons University Library. "Anti-Oppression: Anti-fatmisia." 2024. https://simmons.libguides.com/anti-oppression/anti-fatmisia.

Stoll, Laurie C. "Fat Is a Social Justice Issue, Too." *Humanity & Society*, vol. 43, no. 4, 2019, pp. 421–441.

Stewart, Terah J. "About Fat Campus." *About Campus: Enriching the Student Learning Experience*, vol. 23, no. 4, 2018, pp. 31–34.

Stewart, Terah J. "Course Outlines". Iowa State University, n.d.

Tanner, Anna B. "Unique Considerations for the Medical Care of Restrictive Eating Disorders in Children and Young Adolescents." *Journal of Eating Disorders*, vol. 11, no. 33, 2023.

Tatangelo, Gemma, and Marita McCabe, David Mellor, and Alex Mealey. "A Systematic Review of Body Dissatisfaction and Sociocultural Messages Related to the Body among Preschool Children." *Body Image*, vol. 18, 2016, pp. 86–95.

Wee, Christina C., Ellen P. McCarthy, Roger B. Davis, and Russell S. Phillips. "Screening for Cervical and Breast Cancer: Is Obesity an Unrecognized Barrier to Preventive Care?" *Annals of Internal Medicine*, vol. 132, no. 9, 2000, pp. 697–704.

Wei, Su, and Aurelia Di Santo. "Preschool Children's Perceptions of Overweight Peers." *Journal of Early Childhood Research*, vol. 10, no. 1, 2012, pp. 19–31.

Weinstock, Jacqueline, and Michelle Krehbiel. "Fat Youth as Common Targets for Bullying." *The Fat Studies Reader* edited by Esther Rothblum and Sondra Solovay, New York University Press, 2009, pp. 120–126.

White, Francis R. "Fat/Trans: Queering the Activist Body." *Fat Studies: An Interdisciplinary Journal of Weight and Society*, vol. 3, no. 2, 2014, pp. 86–100.

3

CHOOSING FAT?

INTRODUCTION

If, as the previous chapter asserts, living in a fat body is hard, this chapter seeks to look at the origins of fatness: how it arrives on the body and what may be done to remove it. In the popular imagination, fat is seen as entirely due to personal choices and, as a result, as a self-inflicted site of stigma. This chapter seeks to trouble that assumption by considering the many different inputs which result in fatter or thinner bodies. Acknowledging that fat is complicated and arrives and leaves for many reasons, however, can merely shift the tone from scorn toward pity. Instead, this chapter will trouble the notion of "choice" in the first place, suggesting that no matter why given bodies are fat, they never deserve scorn, pity or stigma. The overwhelming impact of the weight loss industry in the modern era is key to this discussion and will be explored in some detail.

This chapter is framed by the following questions:

- Is being fat a choice?
- What are the consequences of thinking about fat as a choice?
- What is the role of the weight loss industry in framing the idea of choice?

It is impossible to consider size as a site of oppression without delving into the issue of choice. Why are fat people fat? Why are we, as a species, fatter than we used to be, especially in North America? What are the different personal and social reasons why

DOI: 10.4324/9781003539773-3

bodies might assume the range of shapes that they have? Of course, we tend not to ask these questions about natural variations that are seen as relatively neutral, such as height, or even those that are charged but seen as unambiguously genetic, such as race. So many of the nasty traits associated with fat are attached to this idea of choice and bigger issues of how we believe all people should act to be functional members of society. In a modernist society we are committed to the idea of self-determination. Our values and our policies are guided by ideas such as "pulling ourselves up by our bootstraps" or "faking it until we make it". It is therefore unsurprising that most societies in the so-called developed world are informed by rampant workaholism, eating distress, crises of anxiety and stress and enormous disparities in social class. We may be faking it, but we certainly aren't making it. Some of the anxiety around self-determination—as opposed to structural analyses such as looking at the social determinants of health—results in the demonization of fat people. To uncouple fat from choice, however, does nothing to address the major anxieties which underpin our collective commitment to choice, our beliefs that we can and *should* control the outcomes of all aspects of our lives. This chapter will aim to consider some of the ways that fat may or may not be a choice, but will also seek to question whether asking about choice is fruitful, or may be harmful in and of itself.

IS FAT A CHOICE? MAYBE "YES"?

The common sense understanding of fat is found in the popular notion of "calories in, calories out". In other words, fat is seen as simple and universal: all bodies work the same way, and burn fuel at the same rate. To reduce size, simply burn more fuel than you are consuming. This belief suggests that changing food habits (whether they are called diets or "lifestyles"), paired with attention to exercise, can transform a body.

As most people of all sizes know, this belief system may be true in the shortest term—diets can result in rapid short-term weight loss, and changing to different exercise regimes may reduce fat and also change shape and re-arrange muscle mass. That said, bodies work in a range of different ways, burning fuel in different configurations. As will be considered below, not all bodies are able to move in the same ways, for a range of different physical and social reasons. Our metabolisms are variable and dependent on genetics and environment. Furthermore, the short term changes to our body's function can sometimes result in longer term difficulties with burning calories—dieting can actually slow down our metabolisms.

The mainstream belief, however, is that while some people may need to work harder than others, fundamentally, with sufficient willpower, all bodies can change. This issue is less about fat than it is about control: our societal commitment to control is rooted in colonization and white supremacy. Joy is seen as suspicious and all aspects of life—bodies, but also parenting, hobbies, movement—require labour and intensity. This is a very exhausting way to live, in which leisure is punished and even "self-care" is weaponized into work.

All bodies change over the course of the lifespan. Ideally, we grow as young people and illness, reproduction, environment, and many other factors change our shape and size. Our bodies are deeply mutable but on the whole, not within our control, and when we aim to control them anyway, we often do so in ways that present challenges to our physical and emotional health.

Of course, there are some people for whom willpower—of some description—is sufficient to ensure a reduction in size. While not all bodies can ever achieve thinness, some people are able to—or unable not to—control eating to an extent that can result in thinness, sometimes to the point of starvation. The hyper control of extreme eating distress, however, cannot be said to be a health-seeking behaviour. This is, unsurprisingly, the predictable outcome of a non-stop focus on numbers in a climate that valorizes control: counting of calories and minutes of exercise and over-vigilance about the body's functions is a distorted form of control. Where does dieting become eating distress? We tend to pathologize people who are struggling with extreme eating distress, but applaud very similar or the same behaviours when they don't immediately lead to dire physical outcomes. If we take up this view, then perhaps fat is a choice, but the "ability" to control fat comes at an overwhelming cost.

IS FAT A CHOICE? PERHAPS NOT

The overwhelming belief that our bodies are within our control is so widely held and so deeply rooted that it is astonishingly difficult to unseat. Often when I speak about fat as a natural variation outside of our control, I feel like I am suggesting the earth is flat. Despite the pervasiveness of this belief, however, it does not withstand closer attention. Below, I discuss some of the reasons why it may be an error to think of fat as something people can control or choose:

- Fatness is, like most things, overwhelmingly multifactorial. Everyone knows anecdotally about the thin friend who eats more than everyone else and the fat person who seems to live on celery and stays fat. On the whole, attempts to achieve thinness where it does not naturally exist overwhelmingly fail. Given the abundance of evidence on how poorly fat people are treated, if there were a way for fat people to become thin, there would be no more fat people. Unfortunately, the truth of the matter is much more complicated.
- Diets almost always fail. Whether they are fad diets such as grapefruit and cottage cheese, or informed by the "science" of calories in, calories out, on the whole our bodies want to stay at their set point (Hall and Guo 2017) rather than transforming by our will. While many claims are made about the efficacy of various diets, 95% of people who diet regain the weight—and often more—within five years (Mann and Tomiyana 2007). Part of the reason that the weight loss industry is so very lucrative is that there is no form of reliable long term weight loss.
- On the whole, people who diet end up yo-yo dieting, with thousands of pounds lost and gained over a lifetime. The metabolic implications of radically see-sawing between styles of eating are not fully understood, but scholars surmise that a body that is put into starvation mode may compensate by holding stubbornly to weight in the face of future diet attempts (Garvey 2022). Many of the health conditions associated with high weight may be due to the strain on bodies of constant changes in input.

- Our bodies want to eat! Cotugna and Mallick (2010) designed a study for nutrition and dietician students, who are often notoriously fatphobic, measuring their feelings about fat people before and after engaging in a low calorie diet. Many of the students failed to complete the diet, citing that they were too hungry to continue. Importantly, the level of disdain and judgment of fat people was greatly lessened after students actually attempted to take on the intervention they were prescribing.

The Biggest Loser. In "After the After: *The Biggest Loser* and Post-makeover Narrative Trajectories in Digital Media" Margaret Hass (2016) explores the impacts of the popular weight loss reality TV show *The Biggest Loser* (2016). Running for 17 years in its original incarnation, this show pits fat people against each other through punishing challenges related to food and movement, and makes fatness a spectacle. Participants usually reveal a tragic back story that has led to their indefensible lifestyle choices. Despite this focus on pathos, the show ultimate measures success solely by numeric criteria, with the maximum pounds lost ensuring victory. Past participants of the show, however, have come forward to discuss the long term impacts on their physical and mental health as a result of the sustained trauma of starvation and punitive exercise. What is the impact of a show like this, that runs across generations of families, on our story about fat, willpower, resilience and trauma?

- Recently, there has been a huge increase in bariatric surgery, appetite management through stomach size reduction. These surgeries come with a host of risks but are often met with rapid weight loss in the period of time following the operation. Even this intervention, however, does not reliably predict long term weight loss though it may predict other health challenges (Garvey 2022).
- Part of the reason why diets fail is that weight is overwhelmingly genetic. Our body composition is largely predicted by our biological origins and much less by what we do. We understand this about other physical conditions such as height—deprivation or other situational factors can cause us to

be more or less tall than our genetic blueprint, but on the whole, children of short parents are unlikely to be professional basketball players. If we all ate the same food and moved precisely the same ways in childhood, we would all end up with different heights. Why is it so hard to believe that the same is true of weight? We understand that our affinities, our talents, our intelligence, our capacities are effected by both nature and nurture: why are so we unwilling to consider the impact of nature on weight? Molecular geneticist Jeffrey Friedman (2004) writes,

The commonly held belief that obese individuals can ameliorate their condition by simply deciding to eat less and exercise more is at odds with compelling scientific evidence indicating that the propensity to obesity is, to a significant extent, genetically determined. The herit- ability of obesity is equivalent to that of height and greater than that of almost every other condition that has been studied—greater than for schizophrenia, greater than for breast cancer, greater than for heart disease and so on. Although environmental factors contribute to changes in the incidence of obesity over time, individual differ- ences in weight are largely attributable to genetic factors. So, although the current environment, in which almost everyone has essentially unlimited access to calories, can account for an average weight gain of 7–10 pounds over the past decade in the United States, it is genetics and not the environment that accounts for a large proportion of the marked differences in individual body weight in our population today.

(2004, 563)

- Some of the origins of our genetic destiny occur before we are even born. The uterine environment in which we grow can impact our future size and shape, a concept known as "epi-genetics" (Parker 2014). Unfortunately, instead of reminding us how many different factors go into our body composition, these ideas are used solely to police pregnant people for their choices, often at a time when food, movement and body shape are most fraught.
- Nature and nurture do not cease to matter once we are no longer children. We live in environments and communities.

Environmental toxins, prevalence of food deserts, familial traumas, specific community expectations around food and physique—all of these things impact how our bodies exist and evolve over time. The mobility of populations may also have an impact as our access to different environments changes. Are school lunches provided? Do we have time for a coffee break allocated in our day? Does the retirement residence care that we hate cauliflower? The idea that we have choice over how our bodies fit into the world is laughable. Even if the simple calories in/calories out logic were accurate—which is it not— most of us have little to no control over either—yet parents, and specifically mothers, are still given blame for their children's size (Boero 2009)

- Pervasive hatred can change our bodies. If, as established in Chapter 2, living in a larger body causes much pain and even fear of fat can impact our psyches greatly, some of the impact may exist within our metabolic structures, resulting in unexpected changes to our bodies or a resistance to changes we may be trying to enact. These changes may be even more pervasive if we live in the face of multiple different forms of oppression.

- Finally, the impact of poverty cannot be underestimated. Bodies resist being beaten into control, but to even make the attempt requires enormous resources. Access to fresh food, time to make meals, leisure time in which to exercise or otherwise move the body, and the mental space in which to control all these things—these are not equally distributed. In the present moment, the prevalence of expensive weight loss drugs such as Ozempic and Wegovy exacerbates the problem—people with resources will have access to (temporary) thinness, while those without these resources will only be further punished for their seeming lack of control.

WHAT IS THE IMPACT OF ASKING ABOUT CHOICE?

It would seem that asking about how we become or stay fat could help fat people—if we aren't responsible for own "failings" perhaps we will be treated better. While much of the discourse of choice is rooted in good intentions, unfortunately the reality is more complicated.

Generally speaking, we ask whether human differences are rooted in choice in order to discern whether we should offer blame or pity. If fat people are just lazy slobs, then we are "allowed" to hate them—if they're unfortunate schlubs, we must merely feel sorry for them. The premise of the question is rooted in the idea of fat as inevitably and always bad. We don't ask whether people have a choice about their shoe size; we don't ask about the origins of perfect pitch. As LeBesco writes, we seek explanation for conditions that are viewed as problematic or less-than (2009). LeBesco frames the chronology of research around the "gay gene" and the "fat gene" as examples of "fact"-finding rooted in judgment.

As with many other human differences, fat may or may not be a choice for different people at different places and times. Suggesting that fat is multifactorial does not eliminate the role of human agency. Some people identify as "gainers"—people who are deliberately seeking to become as fat as possible (Adams and Berry 2013). While the logic of "calories in/calories out" is imperfect, there is an element through which some of us may control some part of our weight profile, some of the time. In other words—perhaps fat *is* a choice, at least sometimes.

The problem with the conversation about choice is that it suggests a hierarchy of fat life in which only blameless fat folks deserve to be treated with dignity and respect. Some fat people are fat because of underlying health conditions such as Polycystic Ovarian Syndrome. Some fat people have mobility differences that limit capacity for movement. Some people are fat because they live in food deserts or work three jobs or have back-to-back pregnancies. Some people are fat because they eat a lot of food. Some people are recovering from eating distress and refusing to monitor intake as part of their recovery. Fat is complex and so is our relationship with our bodies. There is no singular reason why fat arrives, nor why it sometimes leaves—many people become suddenly thin because of cancer and are lauded for their "healthy" choices. The same way there is no right way to be a human being, there is no right way to be a fat human being and being "well behaved" cannot be a pre-condition for being treated humanely.

Fat Studies scholarship begins from the premise that the human species includes bodies of all sizes, for all reasons, and that all of those bodies are worthy of respect, dignified medical treatment and chairs, among other things. Beginning to organize human behaviours into categories of more or less worthy is unsettling and creates tests that only lead to failure.

IMPACT OF THE WEIGHT LOSS INDUSTRY

The weight loss industry, including diets, bariatric surgeries, weight loss drugs, exercise plans, personal training, etc., is a 90 billion dollar enterprise (LaRosa 2024), and it has only increased its scope and earnings in the last thirty years. It is tempting to believe that the increased focus on weight loss and body management more generally is just a natural trend of human behaviour that happens to have been monetized, but the truth is more insidious: Diets are not increasing because people are getting fatter and sicker. Rather, we are being told that people are fatter and sicker precisely to ensure that the weight loss industry is more lucrative.

Stoll explains the origins of the "obesity epidemic" here:

> While efforts to pathologize and medicalize fat began decades earlier, it was in the early 1980s, when a small group of health professionals, government health officials, and lobbying groups, with ample support from the pharmaceutical and weight-loss industries, began diligently promoting the idea that "obesity" was a disease. Their efforts would start to pay off in the following decade, beginning in 1993 when a study by McGillis and Foege titled "Actual Causes of Death in the United States," was published in the *Journal of the American Medical Association* (*JAMA*). The McGillis and Foege article suggested that a poor diet and a sedentary lifestyle were associated with 300,000 deaths per year in the United States. This study became a major justification for Surgeon General C. Everett Koop to launch the Shape Up America! Campaign (a campaign Weight Watchers, SlimFast, and Jenny Craig contributed over a million dollars to) and declare the war on obesity in 1995. In the same year, the World Health Organization (WHO) issued a report recommending that "overweight" be established at a BMI of 25. The International Obesity Taskforce (IOTF) had a major hand in drafting this report. But as Oliver points out in *Fat Politics*, what most laypeople did not realize was that the IOTF was primarily funded by Hoffman-La Roche, makers of the diet drug Xenical, and Abbott Laboratories, makers of the diet drug Meridia.
>
> (Stoll 4–5)

The weight loss industry would not be as successful if diets worked. If any weight loss plan was a singular, effective and finite intervention, then this industry would fail to be so spectacularly lucrative. Instead, the entire industry is premised on two factors: that bodies left in their natural state are usually deeply flawed and headed toward terrible outcomes (namely death); and that body management is endless and lifelong (which is another way of saying that all diets fail). Simply put, if we are satisfied by our bodies—regarding our looks or our health or both—we do not spend as much money trying to change them.

Even for people not actively engaged with weight management—not enrolled in Weight Watchers, not tracking food intake on their phones—the beliefs offered by the weight loss industry inform daily activities. The omnipresence of nutrition labelling, food pyramids and other tools results in a system where diet talk is pervasive and taken for granted. We are seduced by "expert" knowledge, and the many different forms of expertise that have been funded by the weight loss industry have become canonical truths that are hard to shake.

In some Fat Studies and fat activist spaces, the diet industry is compared to conversion therapies (Bergen and Mollen 2019) for queer and trans people and a broader set of industries such as applied behaviour analysis (ABA) for autism, and even child protection scrutiny, which require the person and family to fit themselves into the environment rather than finding fault with the systems that govern us. In the face of any kind of rampant discrimination there are largely two choices: change the body, or change the environment. In regard to many identity issues, the idea of changing the body is generally seen as problematic: while we engage in behaviours such as accent management and skin whitening, we may also acknowledge that fundamentally these behaviours are apologetic, rather than affirming. Likewise, shame may keep us in various closets—but, at least in progressive spaces, we aim to support the emergence from these states, not to push folks further into their closets. With weight, even in very progressive spaces there may still be a tacit acknowledgment that body management is not only accepted but inevitable. Rather than meeting fat discrimination with affirmation, the body is constantly seen as the source of the problem, and therefore the solution is to change the body. That the body likely can't and won't change is handily overlooked.

The social model of disability (Oliver 2013) suggests that disabled bodies are not flawed or deficient, but rather that the environment fails to meet the range of needs humans embody. Fat studies scholars have extended this analysis to weight (Meleo-Erwin 2014; Herndon 2021) by considering that fat bodies are naturally part of the human landscape and that the limitations imposed upon them are thus structural rather than individual. This is an important idea but one that as yet doesn't have mainstream traction—the overwhelming common sense knowledge is that fat people do not fit because they choose not to.

I am often reminded that other expert discourses have had similar primacy to expert beliefs about fat: "science" believed in the fundamental wrongness of queer and trans folks; "experts" published information on different intelligences based on race—these knowledges have been debunked and are no longer accepted as fact. Furthermore, these forms of knowledge were equally informed by white supremacy and capitalism, the same values which underpin the weight loss industry. Fat Studies asks us to maintain scepticism and to consider that the current belief systems are not innocent and not necessarily true, ideas that will be explored further in Chapter 4 in consideration of fat and health.

You might believe that you live outside of the weight loss complex. There are some questions that you might want to ask yourself: When is the last time I ate whatever I wanted? When is the last time I engaged in exercise even though I didn't feel like it? How do I feel emotionally and cognitively when I eat fruits and vegetables? How do I feel when I eat fries and a burger? The hierarchy of good foods and bad foods, good movement and non-movement, good lives and bad lives is deeply engrained and it's virtually impossible for any of us to escape it. This shouldn't be a reason to feel more guilty—that is completely contrary to the spirit of Fat Studies and fat activism! Rather, I hope to make the reasons why we engage in many different behaviours more transparent in order to start to heal and treat ourselves with greater kindness.

BIOPOWER

The concept of biopower originates in the work of Michel Foucault (1990). Foucault considered the ways that states may control or govern the lives of citizens through impacting biological and physical behaviours. Biopower manifests in two major ways. First, by measuring and controlling individual behaviours through systems of discipline and record-keeping—systems such as BMI measurement in schools, growth charts at doctor's offices and nutrition labelling all place responsibility on individual actors to maintain "normalcy". The second way that biopower occurs is at a population level, gatekeeping access to fertility systems and other treatments, allowing for specific populations to flourish and others to struggle. The impact of biopower is population control, in the sense of literally controlling the population to push societies, as well as the bodies within them, into specific shapes. Meleo-Erwin writes that "Within a system of biopower, in which the focus of governance is on the health and vitality of the population, normalization operates through practices of division, classification, ordering and identification." (2014, 390). By implicating the individual into the responsibility of the health of the nation, biopower demands obedience which is often enacted through shaming and blaming approaches.

There is a great degree of self-regulation of the population in the present day, around and beyond issues of weight. Perhaps more importantly, the idea that we have choices, and that we are therefore responsible for (seemingly inevitable) outcomes of those choices, informs how we live and how we relate to one another. What if we learned from Fat Studies to reject biopower and instead acknowledge that many choices are constrained, especially (but not only) in the area of weight management? What if instead of encouraging docility we truly embraced diversity, both of different shapes and sizes, and of the conditions that create them? Such an approach would respond to Foucault's thinking around the need to reject the regimented and controlling approach of the state and instead thicken our ways of being and relating to one another.

Foucault argues that biopower is "an explosion of numerous and diverse techniques for achieving the subjugation of bodies and the control of populations" (1990, 140). The rationale for why bodies and populations require control is complicated. Social control encourages efficiency and obedience; free will and empowerment are messy. It will never be as cost-effective to make sure that there are chairs for every type of body, and yet in order to create a just society we must truly acknowledge the full range of bodies and behaviours.

MEDIATED BODIES

This chapter necessarily considers some of the ways that every person engages in body management practices. It is virtually impossible to feed ourselves without being informed by the discursive noise about food. We all have a range of reasons why we may or may not move our bodies. These decisions live amongst innumerable others—to wear a dress or pants, to get that tattoo, to stop using that hair straightener, to get the cane. No body goes out into the world unmediated. We all make choices about how we want our bodies to be received and the choices we make, or don't make, around weight, need to be considered within a larger politic where we decide how we want to be seen and understood by the world around us.

In order to think about mediated bodies we need to really break down the idea of choice altogether. There are no choices that we make about our bodies that occur in isolation. When we're put in a pink or a blue sleeper before we have language we're already being put into systems of signification that impact the rest of our lives! In a world that is so overwhelmingly discriminatory toward most people for one reason or another we are constantly navigating how we show ourselves. For example: the "right" outfit for Pride might not be safe for the commute to the march. The clothes I wear for school pickup may not be appropriate when I am teaching a class. Even when these rules are "broken"—there is sometimes an aesthetic of sort of aggressive underdressing in specific spaces including the university—they are deliberately and thoughtfully broken. *We are not allowed not to care.*

Exploring other body choices may help us explain: I am a brown woman with very curly hair and I was taught from a very young age to make sure that my hair was tamed and contained. One of my earliest memories is of my mother putting my hair painfully onto massive rollers and sitting me under a huge hair dryer that looked like the helmet of a spacesuit. I began using chemical straighteners to tame my curls when I was 11. As a young adult I discovered feminism and anti-racist movements and began to embrace my ethnicity in new ways. At 30 I finally stopped using chemical straighteners (the "creamy crack"—if you know, you know) and let my curls emerge. Yet now, in my late forties, I still do not move in the world with unmediated hair. I do not force my children to tame their curls into straight(ish) lines, but I do insist that their hair is tidy, fearing the censure aimed at me as their racialized mother. I twist my curls, use lots of hair goo, do my best to ensure that my hair, and my children's hair, looks "safe" for a world that still aims to disappear someone like me. I offer this example because the continuum of mediated to unmediated bodies is not binary: we do not learn shame, start to engage in body controlling practices, and then become enlightened and stop. Rather, we are engaged in constant negotiation and risk assessment.

Roxane Gay resists the orthodoxy of many fat activist spaces. Instead of cheerily loving her fat, she suggests that living in a multiply Othered body as a tall, fat Black queer woman can be exhausting and overwhelming. While critical of the idea of fat as a choice, she nonetheless writes in her 2017 memoir *Hunger* about some of the deliberate ways she aimed to increase her body size following sexual abuse. In "What Fullness Is: On Getting Weight Reduction Surgery", she also writes about the choice to reduce fat, explaining why she is opting for gastric bypass surgery. These perspectives challenge the usual Fat Studies story of a reformed fatty who now embraces their fat and never intervenes with their body again. Yet Gay's ideas are also familiar to so many people: for most of us the decision to understand more information about fat and fatness can't totally counter a lifetime of weight stigma. We may choose safety and a simpler life even if we know that, for example, diets will only help us temporarily.

As the example above shows, the landscape of decision making around our bodies is hugely complex, in the realm of fat and beyond. We never make any choice about our bodies without a decision making matrix informing what we do. It's a hard world in which to be Other. In the face of the deluge of information we all receive about fat as not only wrong, but also shameful and humiliating, is it any wonder that most of us cannot easily and wholeheartedly reject all body modifying lifestyle choices? In the realm of weight, we may not be ready to give up our body controlling practices. I remember a research participant who said something like "I don't know if I want to be in the project because I won't be able to continue my bulimia if I keep learning about all of this." Controlling ourselves is exhausting and harmful, but in the face of a world that seeks to constantly reduce and eradicate fat people (and all people who deviate from the mythic white male straight norm), it can be easier to give in than give up.

We may seek out spaces that allow us to be common, or usual— even if these moments of respite are brief. I think about the brilliant work of Crystal Kotow (2024) who describes BBW bashes, weekend long retreats for super fat women and their admirers:

> I have been to several bash pool parties over the last four years and they are always spaces where I feel free in my body. They are also always experiences that make me think about how great it would be if I could go to any pool party and feel that comfortable in my body. One of the most fascinating elements of bashes is how they work to normalize fat bodies as a result of exposure to other fat bodies experiencing freedom and joy. I am not concerned about whether I am going break a chair. I am not concerned that I am being judged for my food choices when I'm out with bash friends having dinner before that night's dance. I am not hyperaware of being winded after taking stairs. I can assume that if someone is showing interest in me, it is genuine. In these important ways, I am able to relax into my body and get a glimpse of what it is like for non-fat people navigating their day-to-day lives.

(2024, 153)

Part of what makes these spaces so radical is that the goalposts of "normal" are shifted—miles of exposed fat flesh are expected and appreciated, rather than rejected. At the same time, even in BBW spaces, as Kotow documents, people compare diet tips and engage in competitive exercise conversations.

In our joy at finding fat affirmation, we may want to scold or school fat people who continue to try to change. Yet to do so is not the way to truly embrace fat positivity. At its worst, fat activism and fat affirming spaces can reject one "right" way of living and simply replace it with another. Learning to love your fat so you can jeer at someone who is still participating in diet culture does not result in the transformed world of our dreams. Rather, we must resist fat shaming discourses individually and structurally, but we must also offer compassion about how hard it is to step off the weight hating train. There is no right way to recover from fat phobia, any more than there was a right way to have a body in the first place. Instead, at its best, Fat Studies and fat activist spaces encourage transparency and dialogue, a capacity for critical thinking that fits fat into a larger landscape of perfectionism that is about controlling people and populations. We seek to reject these structures but we also acknowledge their reach and so we offer gentleness as we all navigate a fundamentally difficult world. To do otherwise is to simply re-entrench a new shiny picture-perfect Right Way that we may all fall short of.

Mischel's Marshmallows: In 1970, a psychologist named Walter Mischel undertook an experiment. Based on his anecdotal observations of his children's classmates, he hypothesized that self-regulation could be seen as a predictor for future success and then designed an experiment to prove his idea (Mischel 2014). The research design was relatively simple: young children were left alone in a room with a marshmallow or other delicious treat. They were told that they could eat the treat immediately, but that if they could wait, they would receive two sweets instead of one. The results varied wildly, both in terms of how long children could resist temptation, and also in what resources they drew upon to help themselves. The children were then followed over many years with stunning results: the kids who had managed to hold off the longest were successful across most traditional measures: better academic outcomes, higher test scores, better access to employment and promotion. The conclusion (which was recently debunked) was that capacity for self-regulation helps people succeed.

But what if we chose to come to a different conclusion? What if what Mischel was measuring was conformity, and what if conformity and control are not what allow for the most livable life, but are rather what are most rewarded? The tight control required by all of us to "succeed" may come at very high costs in terms of mental and physical health and overall wellness and access to joy If the measure wasn't, for example, SAT scores, but rather happiness ratings, would the outcomes of this experiment vary? If we made livability and truly nourished and healthy people, families and communities the goal, what would we value?

We have not merely been taught that thin is good and fat is bad. Rather, we have been taught that control is good, that we have total free will and must use it to bully ourselves into submission at all times. That is the measure of a successful life—obedience and conformity. Thinness is thus the side effect, not the malady. And of course—obedience is not merely a way to ensure success, but for many people the only way to avoid negative consequences. For Black children, hyper obedience may be the only way to avoid punishment. For queer and trans folks, being compliant and pleasant may minimize negative interactions. Where is our "choice" in the face of these consequences? Similarly then, in the realm of fat, we may believe we must "choose" to be thinner—even though our actual control of our bodies is very limited—in order to perform obedience. If you can't change the weight, at least you can perform "good fatty"—one who is at least trying follow the rules, even if the rules are impossible and nonsensical.

NEXT STEPS

We can't really think about fat life in the landscape of oppression and justice without confronting the question of why people are fat. If many other areas of discrimination such as race and disability are seen as outside of our control, then what business do we have defending fat people? There is a lot of anger and scorn aimed at fat activism as the height of absurd political correctness. In truth, however, as this chapter has shown, the question of fat as a personal choice is much more complex. Most people cannot control their body size in any significant way for any significant length of time. Perhaps more importantly, however, to ask whether fat is a choice is to immediately agree with the idea that fat equals bad.

This chapter has sought to frame fat as a natural human variation like any other, and to suggest that the devaluing of fat life explored in Chapter 2 is never justified. The hierarchy of good and bad fatties (Bias 2014) does not lead to fat liberation. Rather, in thinking about fat and beyond fat, obedience can't be the price we pay for respect and humane treatment.

Questions about fat as a choice live within a larger system of social constructions about free will, agency, personal responsibility and beyond. This chapter has aimed to demonstrate that our overwhelming hyper-focus on weight is part of a larger system of social control that is limiting the ability of most people to achieve a livable life. The fact that these ideas may seem so radical—that fat bodies, and all bodies, need not maintain nonstop vigilance in order to receive respect—is evidence of how completely we have been programmed into believing that fat is bad, and that it's the responsibility of all of us to remove it.

Of course, there is a lingering elephant in the room as we take up this idea of choice. The endless rhetoric of the obesity epidemic does not merely suggest that fat people are ugly and unseemly. Rather, the language of the obesity epidemic grew alongside an overwhelming health anxiety that is used to control populations in a range of different ways. Simply put, we are committed to cheating death and attempting to control our fat is positioned as one major way to stay alive. It is impossible to think about fat, and about fat and choice, without confronting our concerns about health. The next chapter will thus take up the biggest question facing fat people and Fat Studies: is fat unhealthy?

FURTHER READING

Boero, Natalie. "Fat Kids, Working Moms, and the 'Epidemic of Obesity': Race, Class, and Mother Blame." *The Fat Studies Reader*, edited by Esther Rothblum and Sondra Solovay, New York University Press, 2009, pp. 113–119.

Chalklin, Vikki. "Obstinate Fatties: Fat Activism, Queer Negativity, and the Celebration of 'Obesity.'" *Subjectivity*, vol. 9, no. 2, 2016, pp. 107–125.

Elliot, Charlene D. "Big Persons, Small Voices: On Governance, Obesity and the Narrative of the Failed Citizen." *Journal of Canadian Studies*, vol. 41, no. 3, 2007, pp. 134–149.

LeBesco, Kathleen. "Quest for a Cause: The Fat Gene, the Gay Gene and the New Eugenics." *The Fat Studies Reader*, edited by Esther Rothblum and Sondra Solovay, New York University Press, 2009, pp. 65–74.

WORKS CITED

Adams, Tony E., and Keith Berry. "Size Matters: Performing (Il)Logical Male Bodies on FatClub.com." *Text and Performance Quarterly*, vol. 33, no. 4, 2013, pp. 308–325.

Bergen, Martha, and Debra Mollen. "Teaching Sizeism: Integrating Size into Multicultural Education and Clinical Training." *Women & Therapy*, vol. 42, nos. 1–2, 2019, pp. 164–180.

Bias, Stacy. "12 Good Fatty Archetypes." stacybias.net, June 14, 2014.

Boero, Natalie. "Fat Kids, Working Moms, and the 'Epidemic of Obesity': Race, Class, and Mother Blame." *The Fat Studies Reader*, edited by Esther Rothblum and Sondra Solovay, New York University Press, 2009, pp. 113–119.

Cotugna, Nancy, and Anum Mallick. "Following a Calorie-Restricted Diet May Help in Reducing Healthcare Students' Fat-Phobia." *Journal of Community Health*, vol. 35, no. 3, 2010.

Foucault, Michel. *The History of Sexuality, Volume I: An Introduction*. Translated by Robert Hurley, Pantheon Books, 1990.

Friedman, Jeffrey M. "Modern Science versus the Stigma of Obesity." *Nature Medicine*, vol. 10, no. 6, 2004, pp. 564–569.

Garvey, W. Timothy. "Is Obesity or Adiposity-Based Chronic Disease Curable: The Set Point Theory, the Environment and Second-Generation Medication." *Endocrine Practice*, vol. 28, no. 2, 2022, pp. 214–222.

Gay, Roxane. *Hunger: A Memoir of (My) Body*, Harper, 2017.

Gay, Roxane. "What Fullness Is: On Getting Weight Reduction Surgery." *Medium*, 24 April, 2018.

Hall, Kevin D., and Juen Guo. "Obesity Energetics: Body Weight Regulation and the Effects of Diet Composition." *Gastroenterology*, vol. 152, no. 7, 2017, pp. 1718–1727.

Hass, Margaret. "After the After: The Biggest Loser and Post-Makeover Narrative Trajectories in Digital Media." *Fat Studies: An Interdisciplinary Journal of Weight and Society*, vol. 6, no. 2, 2016, pp. 135–151.

Herndon, April. "Law, Identity, Co-Constructions, and Future Directions." *The Routledge International Handbook of Fat Studies*, edited by Cat Pausé and Sonya Renee Taylor, Routledge, 2021, pp. 88–101.

Kotow, Crystal. *The Hidden Lives of Big Beautiful Women*, Palgrave, 2024.

LaRosa, John. "U.S. Weight Loss Industry Grows to $90 Billion, Fueled by Obesity Drugs Demand." *Market Research Blog*, 6 March 2024, https://blog.marketresearch.com/u.s.-weight-loss-industry-grow s-to-90-billion-fueled-by-obesity-drugs-demand.

LeBesco, Kathleen. "Quest for a Cause: The Fat Gene, the Gay Gene and the New Eugenics." *The Fat Studies Reader*, edited by Esther Rothblum and Sondra Solovay, New York University Press, 2009, pp. 65–74.

Mann, Traci, A. Janet Tomiyana, Erika Westling, Ann-Marie Lew, Barbra Samuels, and Jason Chatman. "Medicare's Search for Effective Obesity Treatments." *American Psychologist*, vol. 62, no. 3, 2007, pp. 220–233.

Meleo-Erwin, Zoe. "Queering the Linkages and Divergences: The Relationship Between Fatness and Disability and the Hope for a Livable World." *Queering Fat Embodiment*, edited by Cat Pausé, Jackie Wykes, and Samantha Murray, Routledge, 2014, pp. 97–114.

Mischel, Walter. *The Marshmallow Test: Mastering Self-Control*, Little, Brown, 2014.

Oliver, Mike. "The Social Model of Disability: Thirty Years On." *Disability & Society*, vol. 28, no. 7, 2013, pp. 1024–1026.

Parker, George. "Mothers at Large: Responsibilizing the Pregnant Self for the 'Obesity Epidemic.'" *Fat Studies: An Interdisciplinary Journal of Weight and Society*, vol. 3, no. 2, 2014, pp. 101–118.

Stoll, Laurie Cooper. "Fat Is a Social Justice Issue, Too." *Humanity & Society*, vol. 43, no. 4, 2019, pp. 421–441.

4

TOWARD DEATH AND DEBILITY?

INTRODUCTION

Perhaps the ideas which underpin the prior chapters are starting to make sense: fat people truly suffer and are a population worthy of protection from discrimination; fat people may or may not have a choice about being fat but should not be treated poorly regardless. The looming question which lingers, however, is central to any understanding of fat life: Is fat unhealthy? This chapter seeks to respond to this question by both articulating some of the problems with equating fat and poor health and suggesting possible other explanations for health concerns. Perhaps more importantly, however, this chapter seeks to consider why our fear of, and hatred toward, perceived ill health may reveal more about us than just our fear of fat.

This chapter is framed by the following questions:

- Is fat unhealthy?
- What are some of the reasons why some fat bodies may face different health outcomes than thinner bodies?
- Are people obliged to seek health?

It is impossible to talk about fat people in the present moment without speaking to the concerns about health that have been taken for granted as obvious consequences of living in a bigger body. This chapter will seek to examine the origins of the language of "obesity epidemic" and question the conclusions of some of the popular stories about fat and health. The chapter will further

DOI: 10.4324/9781003539773-4

explore some of the impacts of fat stigma, as distinct from fat itself. Finally, this chapter will seek to question the impact of "healthism" and ask why striving for health—for all bodies, but especially for fat people—is a moral imperative.

IS FAT UNHEALTHY? UNCOUPLING THE LINK

It has become a taken for granted truth that bigger bodies—those that fit the Body Mass Index descriptor of overweight or obese or morbidly obese or super morbidly obese—are, by definition, unhealthy. Countless punchlines rest on the assumption that we can gauge someone's health by visual examination of their body. We assume that we know both someone's behaviours (as seen in the previous chapter) as well as their future, just by looking at them. Unfortunately, the predictive value of this visual assessment is about as accurate as palm reading or other forms of fortune telling.

There are plenty of fat people who do not have any health concerns. There are plenty of thinner people with high blood pressure, diabetes, heart conditions or other health conditions that are commonly expected to coincide with obesity. If we would like to know if someone has hypertension, the best measure is to take their blood pressure continuously over twenty-four hours (Sharma et al. 2017). Looking at their clothing size is, by contrast, a terrible measure. If we are concerned about someone's blood sugar, a useful measure would be to take blood and test it, ideally after 12–14 hours of fasting. An ineffective measure is to eyeball their belt size and assume we know. Heart conditions are often quite hard to assess, requiring a range of different diagnostic tools. Counting someone's chins is not among those tools. Simply put, there are many, *many* ways to determine the health of various body systems in the modern age, but a visual examination of the size of a body is *not* one of them. This method fails everyone, because we not only assume fat people are unhealthy, we assume thinner people are always healthy and that they also engage in allegedly health seeking behaviours such as diet management and exercise. Looking at someone's body, however, doesn't tell you anything about what they do, or about how long they'll live.

Some of our anxiety is rooted in a need to avoid death. We would like to believe that we have the capacity to avoid death and debility, but we will all die, no matter what we eat, no matter how much we move. Likewise, all of our bodies will have changed capacities over our lives and only a small amount of that outcome is within our control.

In some cases, the fact of fat can be lifesaving. Many of the conditions of so-called "metabolic syndrome" such as diabetes, hypertension and cardiac symptoms have better outcomes among people who are bigger (Bacon and Aphramor 2011). Across all populations, overweight people have better outcomes than underweight people (Flegal 2005). As we age, fat is increasingly protective: among people over fifty-five, the lowest mortality is among people in the obese category (Bacon and Aphramor 2011).

WHAT IS THE DEAL WITH BMI? BODY MASS INDEX AND ITS HISTORY

The Body Mass Index is the major medical tool used to assess size. The scale takes a person's height in meters divided by their weight in kilograms. The numeric output of this calculation is then placed into distinct categories of underweight, "normal" weight, overweight and obese, and decisions about care are made with these categories in mind. While the application of math and categories gives the impression that BMI is rooted in empirical data, it is fundamentally a deeply flawed measure. There is no measure of weight or size that accurately predicts anything. Researchers at the University of Pennsylvania argue that

> BMI (body mass index), which is based on the height and weight of a person, is an inaccurate measure of body fat content and does not take into account muscle mass, bone density, overall body composition, and racial and sex differences.

> (Nordqvist 2022, para. 1)

In other words: knowing your BMI tells you very little about anything other than the difference between your height and weight.

In 1830 an astronomer named Adolphe Quetelet went on a quest to determine the perfectly normal average man. Using exclusively white, Northern European men, Quetelet envisioned the human mean—"l'homme moyen"—as the exemplar to which all people should aspire, and he created a crude scale based on his data collection. Quetelet was motivated by eugenics, the deeply racist idea of aspiring to human ideals through minimizing perceived outliers. Even Quetelet never thought his data should be used for individual diagnosis (Gordon 2020). Rather, his data presented a nascent form of biopolitics, suggesting that overall population trends should move toward whiter, more male, more able and thinner ideals. Unfortunately for all of us, Quetelet's ideas soon grew to have a life of their own.

In 1867, life insurance companies in the United States began to seek forms of measurement that could quantify risk and organize bodies into different scales for the purpose of determining insurance fees. Beginning from the hypothesis that fatter people were obviously less healthy than thinner people, they happened upon Quetelet's scale as a justification and adapted it for use as a diagnostic tool for assessing clients. Despite the quest for "empirical data", there was a great deal of fluidity in the measurements beings used:

> To go even further, the companies weren't following Quetelet's guidance on what counted as "overweight" or "obese"—they were making the numbers up. [Aubrey] Gordon says that the "overweight" category could fluctuate by 40 lbs (around 18 kg) across different insurance companies. It wasn't until the 1940s that these were standardised, and not until the 1970s that the National Institute of Health in America suggested a guideline scale for categorisation—now known as BMI.
>
> (Gray 2021)

Even the final assessment of BMI categories was unstable. In the face of widespread concerns about obesity rates (largely funded by the weight loss industry, see Stoll 2019), the emphasis on BMI became more entrenched in the 1980s and 1990s. In 1997, the cutoffs for different categories were changed and "millions of people became fat overnight" (Wann 2009, p. xiv). If obesity is an indicator of ill health, did these people's health status immediately change?

A scale designed to celebrate conformity cannot possibly acknowledge human diversity. The eugenic roots of the BMI scale represent the need for a singular "right" body, so unsurprisingly, most bodies are determined to be wrong. There is a high degree of confirmation bias here: at all stages of the development of BMI the assumption that fat equals bad and unhealthy informed its creation. Yet the depth of these assumptions is not due to a huge increase in population weight, nor a massive change in health outcomes—if anything people are living longer than ever before, despite being, on average in North America, ten to twenty pounds heavier than people of the past. This confirmation bias is evident when we consider that weight anxiety is a relatively recent phenomenon. Flegal writes that "A 1969 study found that patients and physicians did not view body weight and weight loss as salient medical problems and considered deviations from weight standards to be almost meaningless" (2023, para. 2). She quotes the Institute of Medicine which states that "Prior to the late 20th century, overweight and obesity were not considered a population wide health risk" (in Flegal 2023, para. 2). In one respect, BMI is an accurate measure: a measure of our increasing demonization of fat people, and our widespread health anxiety, rather than a reliable measure of population or individual health.

BMI is rooted in racist, colonialist and outdated logics of bodies and populations. Its continued application is as nonsensical as going to the dentist for bloodletting or applying leeches. It lives in the realm of fads such as intermittent fasting that are rooted in pseudoscience and are deeply discriminatory and problematic in their application. Yet this measure holds us in its grip almost from birth—the weight and height scales are applied to children immediately and kids who are outliers are disproportionately scrutinized. So many different outmoded ways of thinking and measuring have become laughable in the present day—what has informed our abiding commitment to this scale?

BMI is the darling love child of colonialism and capitalism. We want to organize bodies into right and wrong and control the systems around us; ideally, we also want to make money by doing so. In reflecting anxiety about the "obesity epidemic", the weight loss industry gains huge profits, especially since all interventions are destined to fail, ensuring a population that is effectively held hostage. Our bodies are dynamic and variable, and the BMI does not acknowledge any of that. It hampers our health by suggesting it may be predictive of anything and contributes to the demonization of fat people. Flegal speaks to this concern:

recommendations for universal screening and lifestyle interventions generate an intense focus on BMI categories and weight loss without adequate evidence of long-term improvement in morbidity or mortality. Moreover, they ignore several potential sources of harm. A 1998 New England Journal of Medicine editorial cautioned: "Until we have better data about the risks of being overweight and the benefits and risks of trying to lose weight, we should remember that the cure for obesity may be worse than the condition. The focus on BMI also ignores the possible adverse health effects caused by weight bias in health care leading to health care avoidance. More generally, the emphasis on weight loss contributes to discrimination and the harms of weight stigma.

(Flegal 2023, para. 11)

So where do we go from here? Even doctors are acknowledging the ways that BMI is a crass and ineffective way of organizing people. Yet the confirmation bias that fat is predictive of ill health is maintained. New measures are being developed, to acknowledge muscle to fat ratio, waist circumference, and other forms of categorizing bodies. These measures may increase accuracy of record keeping but they still begin with the premise of fat as always bad. They do not predict our likelihood of higher cholesterol or blood pressure. Our genetic history of diseases such as cancer is far more predictive than any measure that involves weight.

SO: IS FAT UNHEALTHY? ALTERNATE EXPLANATIONS

While fat is a deeply imperfect and imprecise predictor of poor health, even allowing for confirmation bias, there is a lot of information suggesting that fat people do have poorer health outcomes with greater frequency than thinner people. Suggesting that more fat people are unhealthy is not the same as saying, however, that fat is always predictive of poor health, or that a simple visual impression of any person is a substitute for actual diagnostics. In this section, I aim to provide possible alternative explanations for any poorer health outcomes which do occur in larger populations.

• First and foremost, stigma has a negative impact on health. Populations that experience societal discrimination and oppression have poorer health, independent of the impact of discrimination in medical care. For example, Black women in the diaspora (i.e. women who experience racism) have increased rates of breast cancer; genetically, the families of those women in their homelands do not show this same increase, suggesting that it is the impact of lifelong racism that results in increased diagnoses (James et al. 2010). The cumulative impact of lifelong hatred is deadly, contributing to auto-immune disorders as well as stress related conditions such as high blood pressure and cardiac issues. Ironically, in the case of fat people, it is fat which is held responsible for these conditions, rather than fatphobia.

"The minority stress model is a framework that foregrounds the central role of stressors uniquely experienced among members of a minority group, including expressions of violence, stigma, and discrimination targeting the group in question, as potentially salient contributors to poor physical and mental health" (Kia et al. 2021, p. 2). In the context of fat people, we can consider that the daily microaggressions and ongoing mental load of anticipating hostile physical and emotional environments can impact physical and mental health.

• While hatred across the lifespan can contribute to poorer health, there is a much more direct impact in the realm of fatphobic healthcare. Healthcare providers are overwhelmingly judgmental of fatter patients. Wann writes that, "Fat women are a third less likely to receive breast exams, Pap smears, or gynecologic exams, but are no less likely to receive mammograms, which may indicate obstetric/gynecology physicians' hesitation to touch fat patients" (2009, xxi). Fat people are counselled about weight loss at every appointment, with other possible explanations for symptoms routinely dismissed. Diagnostic equipment is not always available for larger bodies, resulting in misdiagnosis or the total absence of diagnosis. Fear of fatphobia in medical settings also makes fat people doctor-averse—avoiding going to the doctor is often not good for people's health.

Ellen Maud Bennett died shortly after being diagnosed with inoperable cancer. Her obituary read, in part: "A final message Ellen wanted to share was about the fat shaming she endured from the medical profession. Over the past few years of feeling unwell she sought out medical intervention and no one offered any support or suggestions beyond weight loss. Ellen's dying wish was that women of size make her death matter by advocating strongly for their health and not accepting that fat is the only relevant health issue." Bennett's death would undoubtedly be counted among the higher number of cancer deaths among fat people, instead of being seen as what it was—a case of medical malpractice due to fat oppression.

- The social determinants of health are well established. Poverty, lack of education, lack of access to health care, social isolation—these are all contributors to poorer health at both individual and population levels. Being fat puts people at risk for all of these conditions. Maintaining a body requires wealth and time—but being fat can make it harder to have or keep a job or an apartment—which predicts poverty. Rather than the physical fact of fat itself, perhaps fat people are more prone to poorer health outcomes because of the impact of stigma in its capacity to limit access to the determinants required for health?
- As discussed above, fat people who have health conditions often correlated with fat such as hypertension and diabetes, may have greater longevity and better outcomes from those conditions (Bacon and Aphramor 2011). If more fat people have diabetes, could it be that these issues are correlated rather than caused by fat? Perhaps evolutionarily, those of us already genetically prone to diabetes, for example, may *also* be prone to fat, rather than the relationship being causal.

If our health was seen as inevitable rather than something that can be controlled, perhaps we would simply learn how to treat conditions without requiring the cycle of shame. We do not know why bodies who engage in identical eating habits have different health outcomes; ultimately what we can control about our health is quite limited. On the topic of control, the illusion of control is contributing to a crisis in mental and physical health. Our health is impacted by innumerable factors and very few are within our control, but we are fed the illusion that if we live "clean" we will live long and well. Yet controlling food and exercise is not without cost—it may deprive us of community or leisure time, it may force us into a punishing relationship with ourselves and our bodies, to the extent of the newest form of eating disorder, orthorexia. The overall impact of self-hatred and endless self-regulation is not what I would consider "health". The wellness industry has weaponized the idea that we are infinitely responsible and as a result, wellness has never been further out of reach.

The organization more-love.org has produced cards to bring to doctors' offices. The cards state: "Please don't weight me (unless it's (really) medically necessary)." The back side of the card provides explanations for why being weighed at the doctor's office may be unnecessary or even harmful. Fat patients may fear bringing these cards to the office and being seen as strident or difficult, especially if they live in the intersection with other health or disability issues. Recently, I encountered a doctor who took the proactive choice to provide these cards herself. The notion of having these cards available to patients at a doctor's office—rather than waiting for people to advocate for themselves in the face of so much fat shame—is radical. For more information go to: https://more-love.org/resources/free-dont-weigh-me-cards/

CONFIRMATION BIAS

Simply put, confirmation bias refers to the idea that we see what we expect to see. In research, confirmation bias occurs when a researcher comes into the work with a pre-existing hypothesis and designs the research study with that perception in mind. All research is guilty of some degree of confirmation bias: researchers are, first and foremost, people, and we design our studies based on our beliefs and values. That said, confirmation bias is a known challenge within research, and researchers are expected to try to minimize its impact.

Confirmation bias is a huge issue in the realm of obesity research (Tomiyama 2018). As can be seen above, the thesis that fat always means unhealthy is relatively recent in the public imaginary, but it has become deeply rooted. Even when this thesis is tested, for example, in the case of better health outcomes for larger people with hypertension and diabetes, these findings are referred to as a "paradoxical outcome"(Bacon and Aphramor 2011), one which is unexplainable in the context of the major thesis, rather than the thesis itself coming under scrutiny. Writing in the *Canadian Medical Association Journal (CMAJ)*, Paradis and Reznick explore the ways that metaphors around weight are threaded throughout medical care settings, suggesting that "these metaphors encourage doctors to evaluate every symptom through a weight-focused lens" (2013, 153). Paradis and Reznick asks us to acknowledge that how we think about fat informs what we find in both research and clinical settings, and that an awareness of bias, akin to that which training practitioners (should) receive around gender, race and sexuality, is necessary to confront pre-existing biases.

What are your implicit associations with fat? If you took the Implicit Association Test, which measures some of the values we hold which may lurk under the surface, what would it reveal about your deeply held views about fat and fat people and their health? When did you learn these ideas? How deeply held are they? What is your emotion when you think about the potential of confronting these beliefs?

There are two major reasons why confirmation bias is so deeply engrained within research and practice with fat people. The first is that research will always reflect the values and biases of the world in which it is undertaken. We are not able to divorce ourselves from common sense understandings. For this reason, queer identities were taken for granted as negative through centuries of psychological and scientific research. Similarly, social "causes" of autism were analyzed and scrutinized before mothers were blamed for their inability to attach to their children—the bias confirming the claim. (Obviously, in the present day, neither queer nor neurodivergent identities should be viewed as anything other than

possible ways of being human and as a result, no blame is required for their origins.) The second, more troubling reason for confirmation bias in obesity research is all about money: the stranglehold of so many weight loss industries, as well as industries rooted in allegedly health seeking behaviours (most often suggesting self-regulation and hyperscrutiny of diet and exercise as the recipe for health) means that research is funded and set up to find what it wants to find (Stoll 2019). For millennia, humans believed the earth was flat. My hope is that we look back at this era with the same sense of absurdity toward our earlier misguided selves.

Katherine Flegal is a senior scientist at the Centres for Disease Control in the United States. Her research has looked at large scale sets of public data around weight that involved millions of people. Importantly, the data that Flegal used was not funded by anyone with ties to the weight loss industry. When she initially undertook this research in 2005 she found that over these large data sets the highest mortality was among people in the underweight category of BMI, with the highest longevity (longest lifespan) among people in the overweight category. She published this data assuming that the field would welcome a course correction on the popular thinking on this topic. Instead, she was subjected to a backlash that has lasted for almost 20 years, even though further research continues to maintain her findings. In "The Obesity Wars and the Education of a Researcher: A Personal Account" she writes that her initial naivete as a researcher meant that she assumed people would just want the truth (Flegal 2021). Instead, she was subjected to misogynist baiting, public scorn and a rejection of her professional credibility. Katherine Flegal is a deeply impressive and highly trained researcher, yet her skills and capacities still did not give her enough clout to contradict the "official" story of fat and health. Her example reminds us of the deep threads of confirmation bias, and the huge financial investment in the fat = death hypothesis. Thinking about fat life differently is not only heresy—it's literally bad citizenship and as a result, it's a bias that is very hard to budge.

CONFIRMATION BIAS IN FAT STUDIES

While the field of obesity studies has real problems with confirmation bias, arguably so too does the field of Fat Studies. Much of the scholarship coming out of Fat Studies spaces assumes that all fat life is good life, that fat bodies cannot, and therefore should not, change. Fat life, however, like all life, is complex and messy. Some fat people may still wish to try to control their bodies, even after learning about some of the ideas covered in this book. Some fat people may never stop wishing they were not fat. Fat Studies can sometimes replicate the same colonial need for certainty and clean lines that is found in the fields it aims to refute. While the best of Fat Studies scholarship aims to complicate fat life and lean into the mess, it can be tempting to replace the idea of an ideal body with an ideal way of being fat. We will not save ourselves from perfection by merely worshipping at a new altar—instead, we must keep challenging ourselves, in Fat Studies spaces and beyond—to reject the idea of perfection altogether and live with the ambivalence and complexity our lives naturally offer.

HEALTHISM

Perhaps even more engrained than the belief that fat contributes to ill health is the belief that health is always good, always achievable and required to be fought for. Yet these beliefs also reveal deeper values and do not always withstand our analysis. Healthism is defined as a focus on health-seeking behaviours as intrinsically the responsibility of all citizens and actors (Metzl and Kirkland 2010). Mackert and Schorb argue that

> Situating the problem of health within the individual shifts the focus from the social to the personal and paves the way for an understanding of health as an issue of individual control and a result of 'good' or 'bad' choices and behavior.
>
> (2022, 3)

Healthism is problematic for a number of reasons. First, the emphasis on health suggests that people who are, for any reason, unhealthy, are less worthy and more flawed. Yet people live

outside of health for a range of reasons—arguably almost every person will experience times of ill health. Some people live throughout their lives with chronic health conditions, others may face precipitous changes in health status. Our health may change as a result of accident or disease. If we are lucky enough to achieve old age, virtually all of us will end our lives unhealthy, almost by definition.

Further, while knowledge can be useful and powerful, the vague sea of knowledge in which we all swim does not provide clear guidance but rather a climate of fear and control. Rather than a focus on reducing harm, we frame health in the context of achieving perfection, and as a result when we inevitably fall short, we immediately ask what went wrong, who screwed up. This inclination is natural—what we're really asking is "How do I stay safe? How do I keep the people I care about safe?"— yet in believing we can answer this question we are harming ourselves and others.

In many religious spaces, there is a quest for morality and obedience that is the threshold expectation for worthiness. By obeying the rules, the idea goes, you will be admitted to Heaven (or its equivalent, depending on your faith system). The belief in good and evil is so taken for granted that for religiously observant people, what may seem nonsensical to the secular is binding and impossible to avoid. Health has, for many people both religious and secular, become equally binding. Health-seeking is the new morality, and any behaviour that is deemed health-avoidant (behaviours that are ultimately impossible to steer clear of, because there are so many and because they often contradict one another) is a sign of sin. LeBesco writes that,

> The fat person who argues moral validity by saying that he can't help being fat and has good eating habits and takes plenty of regular exercise seeks deliverance. It is an understandable goal, but one based on truly fraught reasoning that allows healthism to flourish unchecked.

(2010, 77)

In religious spaces the same questions are asked as above: "How do I stay safe? How do I keep the people I care about safe?" The uncle who prays for your return to heterosexuality as a pathway to your salvation purports to care about your spiritual safety; the well-intentioned parent who does not affirm your gender wants to free you from potential violence. In justice-minded spaces, we have come to understand that the quest for normalcy is not a pathway to safety, at least not much of the time. Yet while celebrating authenticity and rejecting conformity in many critical spaces, the quest for health goes unquestioned—even at the feminist organizing retreat, many of the people are picking the salad they don't want and pushing away the fries.

The suffocating hold of healthism is challenged along many axes, including weight, in the collection *Against Health*, the cover of which provocatively shows a lit cigarette with smoke wafting from its tip (Metzl and Kirkland 2010). What would it look like to acknowledge risk and aim to live a full, joyous, passionate life while acknowledging that health is a receding goal? How would we conceive of "health" if we took into account our social, spiritual, emotional and mental health and aimed to love ourselves unconditionally rather than punishing our physical selves in the name of some kind of "better" living? Healthism requires a "Basics" book of its own and this brief description cannot begin to do justice to such a vast topic, but exploring the health conditions of fat people cannot be undertaken without at least an elementary understanding.

HEALTH AT EVERY SIZE

In some of the earlier formal scholarship on fat, many authors and scholars aimed to posit other more nuanced ways of thinking of fat bodies outside of the obesity witch hunt which characterizes so much contemporary literature and practice. As the examples above demonstrate, the evidence that weight always and inevitably leads to ill health is quite weak, and where high weights are correlated with poorer health outcomes there is a range of possible explanations that push responsibility beyond the simple fact of fat on any given body.

In response to the demonization of fat, a group of critical dieticians, Fat Studies scholars and other researchers presented a new framework for thinking through fat and health: Health at Every Size.

First presented in 2010, HAES was broadly composed of three key ideas:

- The idea of intuitive eating, in which people re-learn how to respond to their bodies hunger cues and desires. This frame suggests that in rejecting some of the "food noise" around us, we might be free to instead allow our bodies to explore food differently, eventually rejecting ideas of good and bad foods and instead just eating what and when we choose.
- HAES suggests that we move toward joyful movement, both celebrating the moving we already might be doing in the activities of daily living, and also aiming to see moving as a something we do in aid of pleasure rather than pain. In this framework, we should seek out the long walk with a friend or folk dancing class or fat swim, rather than doing more cardio reps at the gym with the mean trainer.
- Finally, HAES suggests that we become (somewhat) body activists, refusing to be at war with our own bodies and rejecting the premise that our bodies are failures based on our size. By rejecting the premise of health and weight as inherently linked, HAES asks us to explore the possibilities of living in body neutral ways (Bacon 2010; Bacon and Aphramor 2011).

HAES quickly gained attention and notoriety. Many people in healthcare fields, in particular, sensed that they were harming their clients/patients with mainstream approaches to fat and were eager to embrace an alternative that still centred health but allowed for less of a punitive focus on fat people. HAES has made inroads into spaces that more ambitious fat activism might not have been able to infiltrate. But does HAES truly present radical alternatives?

Lucy Aphramor and Lindo Bacon authored one of the key papers that led to the popularity of Health at Every Size. Published in 2011, the article "Weight Science: Evaluating the Evidence for a Paradigm Shift" considered the flaws in traditional diet science and posited HAES as a credible alternative that divorced health seeking behaviours from the size of the body doing the seeking. In 2021, however, Lucy Aphramor published what essentially amounted to a retraction of the original paper, suggesting that HAES was deeply flawed and did not invite a true rethinking of weight and health paradigms, but instead presented a palatable but still deeply healthist and weight-phobic framework. Responding to the original article Aphramor writes that, "providing inclusive, respectful, culturally competent lifestyle interventions as a means to reduce early death is actually a prescription for social murder camouflaged in a glitzy wrapping of right-on rhetoric." (2021, para. 26)

Two key ideas are essential to the critique of Health at Every Size: first, in maintaining a commitment to health, HAES still suggests that healthy bodies are better than unhealthy bodies, undermining the efforts of disability activists and other critical scholars and activists to consider that all bodies are worthy. Second, HAES insidiously maintains a commitment to individual labour and self-betterment, sneakily affirming the very value system it seeks to disrupt. HAES maintains the idea of conditional human-ity—that only people who follow the rules are "worthy". It seems radical on the face of it by extending humane treatment to larger bodies, but only to bodies who continue to chase health. In doing so, it both maintains a hierarchy of good and bad fatties, but also plays into the health morality and commitment to individual choice and control that Fat Studies (at its best) seeks to disrupt.

NORMATIVE VS. NORMAL

Chrisler suggests that current medical wisdom adheres to the "Goldilocks" rule (2017, 38) which suggests that there are perfect parameters within which all bodies must live. While it is necessary to understand, for example, how fast or slow hearts can beat before they are in crisis or how much iron is necessary for a body to maintain its functioning, other body systems are much less objective. (Even these "objective" measures include variability—babies' hearts beat much faster than those of adults.) In beginning to frame ideas about what constitutes normal or "usual" health, unfortunately we have slid into normativity, suggesting that all bodies should ideally function in the same ways across all axes. This quickly deteriorates into seeing bodies that function differently as fundamentally wrong.

Most humans poop out our buttholes, but people with a colostomy are not failures. Most humans produce insulin but dia-betic people are not freaks. Many people are heterosexuals but the range of other possible sexualities is to be celebrated, not viewed as "abnormal". The focus on health as a narrow and consistent state that is possible across the life cycle is ludicrous and our ceaseless chasing of health is causing an epidemic of stress and anxiety.

What would change in your life if you did not believe that you were responsible for your health *or* your size? What would you do differently on any given day if you could shed that responsibility and instead believe that, to a fairly large extent, your health outcomes and size were predetermined? What would happen if you challenged yourself to live, even for one day, based on intuitive desires, instead of rules and plans? When I've discussed this in public lectures and classrooms people report that this idea feels liberating but also terrifying—we rely on the idea that we can control our health to alleviate our health anxieties in the short term, but we create more anxiety in the long run.

NEXT STEPS

So where do we go from here? To be frank, this was the scariest part of this book to write, because the belief that fat is unhealthy feels immovable, and rejecting it feels like heresy. In all honesty, sometimes I have a hard time remembering that I'm not suggesting the social equivalent of a flat earth—that I have carefully reviewed a wide range of research that supports the idea that health and size are simply not the same thing. Further, I have come to believe, as a former social worker, parent, teacher and human being, that the endless quest for health is *not* keeping us healthy, or well, or whole.

There are two somewhat contradictory premises here—that fat people aren't inherently unhealthy, but also that health itself is volatile, elusive and changeable and as such, is a terrible basis for decisions about who deserves what treatment. I don't mean to underestimate the awful toll of chronic health conditions, especially chronic pain; the stigma of living in a society designed for normative bodies is inescapable, and furthermore some health conditions or disabilities do include experiences of pain or distress themselves. As Eli Clare reminds us, there are nuances of "cure" in which our desires for our bodies to be different may sometimes be as complicated as our bodies themselves (2017). That said, precisely because so much of our experience is beyond our control, we must begin to allow for the full range of our experiences to meet with relational, kind and responsive care.

Some fat people are healthy. Some fat people are unhealthy. All fat people, and people of all health statuses, deserve to have their humanity respected and access to affirming and responsive healthcare. As a people, all of our choices and indeed, the facts, identities and experiences of our lives all occur as a result of a wide range of different factors. Who we are, what we do, how we look are all chaotic and dynamic—we shouldn't be judged by the width of our waists or the narrowness of our arteries.

This chapter may be hard to digest. If it makes you uncomfortable it may be worth considering why. If you love fat people but worry about their wellness, this chapter is for you. If you are a fat person who can't let go and accept yourself because you are worried about your imminent death, this is for you. If you're the parent of a fat child and you are feeling pressure to reject your child's body, this is for you. I don't know how we heal from the rampant fatphobia that surrounds us, but I do know that using health as a weapon does not result in a population that is well and whole.

FURTHER READING

Aphramor, Lucy. "Hey! Are You One of the 401k Readers Misled by Our HAES Theory?" *Medium*, June 30, 2021. https://lucy-aphramor.medium.com/hey-a re-you-one-the-401k-readers-misled-by-our-haes-theory-14bc3b02276e.

Bacon, Lindo, and Lucy Aphramor. "Weight Science: Evaluating the Evidence for a Paradigm Shift." *Nutrition Journal*, vol. 10, no. 9, 2011, pp. 1–13.

Chrisler, Joan C., and Barney, Angela. "Sizeism Is a Health Hazard." *Fat Studies*, vol. 6, no. 1, 2016, pp. 38–53.

Flegal, Katherine M. "The Obesity Wars and the Education of a Researcher: A Personal Account." *Progress in Cardiovascular Diseases*, vol. 67, 2021, pp. 75–79.

Paradis, Elise, Kuper, A., and Reznick, R. K. "Body Fat as Metaphor: From Harmful to Helpful." *CMAJ*, vol. 185, no. 2, 2013, pp. 152–153.

Tomiyama, A. Janet, Deborah Carr, Ellen M. Granberg, Brenda Major, Eric Robinson, Angelina R. Sutin, and Alexandra Brewis, "How and why Weight Stigma Drives the Obesity 'Epidemic' and Harms Health." *BMC Medicine*, vol. 16, no. 123, 2018.

WORKS CITED

Aphramor, Lucy. "Hey! Are You One of the 401k Readers Misled by Our HAES Theory?" *Medium*, June 30, 2021. https://lucy-aphramor.medium.com/hey-a re-you-one-the-401k-readers-misled-by-our-haes-theory-14bc3b02276e.

Bacon, Lindo. *Health at Every Size: The Surprising Truth about Your Weight*, BenBella Books, 2010.

Bacon, Lindo, and Lucy Aphramor. "Weight Science: Evaluating the Evidence for a Paradigm Shift." *Nutrition Journal*, vol. 10, no. 9, 2011, pp. 1–13.

Chrisler, Joan C. & Barney, Angela. "Sizeism is a Health Hazard." *Fat Studies: An Interdisciplinary Journal of Weight and Society*, vol. 6, no. 1, 2016, pp. 38–53.

Clare, Eli. "Nuances of Cure." *Brilliant Imperfections: Grappling with Cure*, Duke University Press, 2017, pp. 53–68.

Flegal, Katherine M. "Use and Misuse of BMI Categories." *AMA Journal of Ethics*, vol. 25, no. 7, 2023, pp. 550–558.

Flegal, Katherine M. "The Obesity Wars and the Education of a Researcher: A Personal Account." *Progress in Cardiovascular Diseases*, vol. 67, 2021, pp. 75–79.

Flegal, Katherine M., Barry I. Graubard, David F. Williamson, and Mitchell H. Gail. "Excess Deaths Associated with Underweight, Overweight, and Obesity." *JAMA*, vol. 293, no. 15, 2005, pp. 1861–1867.

Gordon, Aubrey. *What We Don't Talk about when We Talk about Fat*, Beacon Press, 2020.

Gray, Chloe. "BMI: This Podcast Exposes the History of BMI (and Why It's Really Not Fit for Purpose)." *Stylist*, August 3, 2021.

James, Carla, Wanda Thomas Bernard, David Este, Akua Benjamin, Bethan Lloyd, and Tana Turner. "Racism Is Bad for Your Health." *Race and Well-Being: The Lives, Hopes and Activism of African-Canadians*, Fernwood Press, 2010, pp. 115–140.

Kia, Hannah, Kinnon Ross MacKinnon, Alex Abramovich, and Sarah Bonato. "Peer Support as a Protective Factor against Suicide in Trans Populations: A Scoping Review." *Social Science & Medicine*, vol. 279, 2021, pp. 1–14.

LeBesco, Kathleen. "Fat Panic and the New Morality." *Against Health: How Health Became the New Morality*, edited by Jonathan Metzl and Anna Kirk-land, New York University Press, 2010, pp. 72–81.

Mackert, Nina, and Friedrich Schorb. "Introduction to the Special Issue: Public Health, Healthism, and Fatness." *Fat Studies: An Interdisciplinary Journal of Weight and Society*, vol. 11, no. 1, 2022, pp. 1–7.

Metzl, Jonathan and Kirkland, Anna, editors, *Against Health: How Health Became the New Morality*, New York University Press, 2010.

Nordqvist, Christian. "Why BMI Is Inaccurate and Misleading." *Medical News Today*, January 20, 2022. https://www.medicalnewstoday.com/articles/265215.

Paradis, Elise, Kuper, A., and Reznick, R. K. "Body Fat as Metaphor: From Harmful to Helpful." *CMAJ*, vol. 185, no. 2, 2013, pp. 152–153.

Sharma, Manuja, Karinne Barbosa, Victor Ho, Devon Griggs, Tadesse Ghirmai, Sandeep K. Krishnan, Tzung K. Hsiai, Jung-Chih Chiao, and Hung Cao. "Cuff-Less and Continuous Blood Pressure Monitoring: A Methodological Review." *Technologies*, vol. 5, no. 2, 2017.

Stoll, Laurie Cooper. "Fat Is a Social Justice Issue, Too." *Humanity & Society*, vol. 43, no. 4, 2019, pp. 421–441.

Tomiyama, A. Janet, Deborah Carr, Ellen M. Granberg, Brenda Major, Eric Robinson, Angelina R. Sutin, and Alexandra Brewis. "How and why Weight Stigma Drives the Obesity 'Epidemic' and Harms Health." *BMC Medicine*, vol. 16, no. 123, 2018.

Wann, Marilyn. "Foreword: Fat Studies: An Invitation to Revolution." *The Fat Studies Reader*, edited by Esther Rothblum and Sondra Solovay, New York University Press, 2009, pp. ix–xx.

Wiley, Rachel. "Fat Joke." *Medical Traumas*, December 17, 2018. https://medicaltraumas.wordpress.com.

5

FAT AND POPULAR CULTURE

INTRODUCTION

This book has asked, several times, where we learned our ideas about fat. Like all collective ideas, these are ideas we have been socialized into, by our families, our education, and perhaps most insidiously, through popular culture. In this chapter we explore both the origins of fat phobia in multiple forms of media and also consider sites of resistance.

This chapter is framed by the following questions:

- How are fat people presented in popular media?
- What are some of the common roles that fat characters are assigned?
- What is the impact of fat in the realm of fashion and dress?
- What are some of the ways that fat is reclaimed in popular culture?

This chapter will take up themes of representation, considering the ways that fat people are shown in television, film, books and other media, looking at the ways that fat characters are portrayed negatively or as side characters. Particular attention will be paid to social media as a means of extending representation of fat bodies in both positive and negative ways. The chapter will also consider fat fashion and the ways that clothing is increasingly less available the larger the size.

DOI: 10.4324/9781003539773-5

WHAT DO WE MEAN BY POPULAR CULTURE?

Culture is all around us, and we both create it and also receive it. Often in human services spaces there are notions of "cultural competence" which unfortunately usually translate to "figuring out how to deliver white services to non-white clients"—there are so many assumptions of who is or does what in that framing! I have come to think of cultural competence in a different way: as the act of becoming critical and loving respondents to the many different forms of culture with which we consume and engage. Often we believe that our political, thoughtful and justice-seeking lives are separate from the time we spend watching *The Bachelor* or going to IKEA or reading a cheesy thriller. All of us, however, are inter- acting with the larger culture—and contributing to it—at all times, and becoming critical consumers is essential. Importantly, this does *not* mean feeling guilty for engaging with problematic content. *All* content is problematic, in one way or another. The media around us—popular media, social media, all of it—is a reflection of, and a contributor to, the broader values; our society is racist, sexist, homophobic and profoundly outraged by fat people. If we're waiting for perfect cultural offerings, we're going to need to invent a new culture— and some of the media examined below is part of this revolution. That said—sometimes we just want to watch TV. No one is immune from this and guilt is unhelpful. Rather, this chapter aims to support transparency in exposing some of the more difficult ideas about fat people that are all around us. In so doing, this chapter hopes to help readers become more critical consumers of culture more broadly, so that we can understand how our beliefs are formed and begin to ask harder questions, even as we continue to engage with the media around us.

MAJOR TROPES

Across all forms of media there are specific tropes of fat people that recur. The fat person is seldom the protagonist, but often relegated to the sassy best friend. Fat men are even less common than fat women but both are obviously undesirable (and there are virtually zero portrayals of fat people outside the gender binary). Fat people are undersexed but hypersexual, part of their rampant greediness.

This is especially true in contexts where fat Black women are portrayed; alternately, however, fat Black women are portrayed as abject victims such as in the example of *Precious*. Fat Black women are also made into Aunt Jemimas and Mammies, caregivers whose ample arms can soothe white pain. Fat people with disabilities must be disabled by their fat, rather than any alternate causal pathway. Fat people are always greedy and must engage in binge eating at all times—any food shown or described as being eaten by a fat person must be "bad" food. Fat people do not care about their health or indeed, about much else—they are simultaneously hedonistic and pathetic. That said, fat people, especially fat girls and women, *must* be aware of their fat to the extent of trying to lose weight. Indeed, this trope of body dissatisfaction is so ubiquitous that it is a staple gag of virtually all media that includes women—the slightly more curvaceous friend who is locked into battle with her body. What fat people aren't: doctors, professors, love interests, runners, dancers, successes by any measure. Is it any wonder that from earliest childhood we understand this as a fate we should avoid?

The hypervisibility of fat does make it distinct from other identity categories. Until quite recently there was limited queer representation and virtually no trans representation in any mainstream media. Even now, children can easily grow up never learning that trans people exist unless families go out of their way to ensure that this knowledge is shared. This is obviously especially dangerous for kids who know themselves to be trans but have no basis for this understanding. Likewise, people with disabilities are largely outside of most media with the exception of revolting inspiration porn. Fat people, however, are ubiquitous. While usually kept on the margins of any given narrative there are nonetheless virtually infinite examples of fat people across all kinds of media. We are therefore very aware of fat people and fat life without necessarily ever being presented with a full range of fat possibilities.

For people who grow up fat or who become fat, how do we come to understand ourselves? The whole story about us is one of revulsion and/or pity. We know that love, success, fame, money—all will be denied us. Is it any wonder then, that we try to flee fat—unsuccessfully—at all times? We are sitting ducks for the weight loss industry which neatly colludes with mainstream media to ensure that we are told that shrinking ourselves is the only pathway to "health", but also to anything like a livable life. Examining specific examples of fat characterization in a range of media underscores this thesis.

LITERATURE

Reading to children is an essential part of helping them find their place in society. The expert discourse (which is itself deeply problematic, an analysis that might need to be saved for another book!) suggests that all parents should read to their children beginning in infancy. This, of course, ignores limits of time, literacy, language and other barriers and is problematic in terms of reifying good parenting (by which we mean good mothering ...). That said—many children are exposed to many ideas through books, beginning at very young ages.

Even the most elementary books tend to show normative body types, even when those bodies are not human. The chubby bear or piglet who is also a little dim and clumsy is so ubiquitous that it is difficult to isolate examples. Before children even access language fully they are being absorbed into systems of thinking that present "right" and "wrong" bodies (across many axes including gender and ability and race, but at present I will restrict this analysis to thinking about fat!).

Moving into chapter books, examples of fat children abound. Fat characters are evil, for example, Dudley and Mr. Dursley who are nearly the only fat people within the *Harry Potter* universe. Children reading the book know immediately what kind of child Dudley is because he is fat—greedy, lazy, mean and stupid. Other books present fat characters sympathetically but still as pitiable deviants. In my own childhood the Judy Blume book *Blubber* exemplified this trope by cataloguing the ways that a fat girl is bullied. Importantly, however, this book did not entirely humanize its protagonist and for many of us, stood instead as a cautionary tale of how awful fat life could be. Of course—we already knew that this was the case. Reading L. M. Montgomery's *Anne of Green Gables* I learned at a very young age that the fat friend could only be a sidekick, a punchline, and that the protagonist would need to exemplify both slenderness and cleverness in equal measure. (These ideas are taken up beautifully Emily Bruusgaard's chapter in *Fat in*

Canada which examines fat tropes in *Anne of Green Gables* in detail.) It is astonishingly hard to find a children's book that presents a fat character positively. The few which exist, such as *Starfish* by Lisa Fipps, are stories of reclamation, but the idea of an unremarkable but larger character is virtually non-existent.

As adults these themes are maintained. Fat characters are the villains across all genres of writing and fat people are either entirely absent or are relegated to the margins. "Curvy" protagonists who agonize about their size but are actually revered by their lovers (looking at you, *Bridget Jones*), have come into ascendency but frankly, speak to the ubiquity of all women hating their bodies and seldom present actually fat people. While there is a growing field of fat utopic fiction, especially in romance novels, these books remain outliers that are preaching to the choir— fat people seek out books that may centre their experiences rather than the world at large having an opportunity to think of fat in three dimensions.

MOVIES

Film presents unique possibilities for the presentation of fat life. As a visual medium film may show rather than tell, portraying fat people cruelly and with a focus on the ways that fat bodies may deviate from those around them. Of course, in the cinematic universe the percentages of fatter people are so minute that any person who is even slightly larger than tiny will be, by comparison, viewed as large. Some films present this comparison as automatically and essentially hilarious: Fat Amy in *Pitch Perfect*, for example, is portrayed by the very funny Rebel Wilson, but the key to her personality is in her excess and her audacious confidence, which is only funny because she is fat. *Mean Girls* capitalizes on a similar trope, suggesting that the cruel prank played by the protagonist of convincing her frenemy to eat high-calorie protein bars instead of the diet bars she believes them to be, is a really funny gag. Obviously nothing could be funnier than making a skinny girl fat, and the scenes where she can't buy clothes at a mainstream shop, or can't find anything to wear, are just the hilarious punchline. Other films use fat suits to ensure that the absurdity of fat bodies is displayed in its full freakery—Eddie Murphy's *The Nutty Professor* franchise, for example, is deeply fatphobic. Importantly, the joke almost doesn't have to be told—this is a purely visual gag where a thin man playing a fat man is, alone, meant to be funny. Lest we believe that fat hatred in film is restricted to comedic offerings, the dramatic film *The Whale*, which met with huge critical acclaim, also resorts to the use of a fat suit for its protagonist who is shown as unlovable and abject, a pathetic and calamitous figure with nothing to live for. There seems to be no reflexivity of the fact that the portrayal of fat people (and in the case of *The Whale*, specifically superfat people) as having impossible and unlivable lives may, in fact, be creating the reality it aims to display.

Importantly, the hateful treatment of fat people in film is so omnipresent that it is almost impossible to categorize. These few examples are the tip of the iceberg. The barfing teen in *Stand By Me*, the thunderous impact of *Thor*, who meets depression with corpulence to great laughs—each of these examples contribute to the belief that only pathetic and greedy people are fat and that to be fat is incompatible with a good life—and in telling this story, the story becomes true. We learn that to be fat is horrible and that to fall in love with fat can only be fetish. We learn to run from fat as fast and as hard as we can and when we can't—we know exactly what we deserve. This is a different version of *Mean Girls* in which it is the mythical mean that is causing harm by being mean.

TELEVISION

Growing up in the 1980s and 1990s, so much of my information about the world was informed by television. Even though I wasn't an avid watcher, soap operas were blaring in the background, and even just an awareness of the bodies on talk shows informed my consciousness from a very young age. I noticed, and continue to note, that fat people were and are notably absent from mainstream television.

In the context of sitcoms, fat people are either the sassy sidekick, similar to those in the film universe discussed above, or sometimes the mean alternative. The fat character is almost never the protagonist and in the rare case when this is transgressed, such as in the show *Mike and Molly*, the show revolves around weight. *Roseanne*, one of the first shows to profile a fat couple at its centre, ran through ten seasons of fat jokes and solidified the connection between working class and fat cultures. It is precisely the crassness and poverty of the show's protagonists that situate their fat bodies. It is impossible to imagine a show like *Beverly Hills 90210*—any of its incarnations—showcasing a fat body. Indeed, all of the shows that are set in high schools are notably free of fat characters with the exception of the rare person who is set up as a hilarious foil to the ubiquitous thinness—think Lauren Zizes on *Glee*, for example.

Unfortunately, like movies, sometimes television shows take fat hatred and scorn further. The canonical example of this is on the long running and wildly popular show *Friends*. One of the key characters is revealed to have a secret fat past, portrayed by actor Courtney Cox in a fat suit, generally shown to be stuffing her face. Notably, Fat Monica is a completely different character than Usual Monica—crass, cloying, over eager, hungry in all regards. What does it mean to watch this beloved show and suddenly see a body like yours—a body that, by all accounts, better resembles the majority of North American women!—and know, once again, that you are the butt of the joke? Kent writes:

> Everything from how the character was designed—à la the svelte Courtney Cox in a fat suit rather than an actual person who was, gasp, fat—to how the character acted was greatly exaggerated to elicit laughs—and not much else. In an alternate opening sequence, Fat Monica hops onto the gang's couch and almost tips it over—and we're supposed to laugh. Fat Monica is often seen eating sloppily, wiping chocolate from her face, or licking powdered sugar from her fingers. In "The One That Could Have Been" a two-parter where Monica never loses weight in an alternate timeline, she remains a virgin for the longest time (because *apparently* fat people didn't have sex in the '90s?). And the show plays up the character's hallmark neuroses for laughs when she is overly concerned with someone having sat on her Kit Kat bar (because being neurotic or struggling with OCD is complex ... unless you're fat) in the same episode.
>
> (Kent 2019, para. 4)

For years, many shows had a fat, stupid and often oversexed character. While this trope is withering somewhat, it has been replaced by a resounding absence of fat characters. Is it better to be mocked or erased? What does it do to our brains when virtually all bodies that are in the public space look a very specific way—usually white, predominantly within the gender binary, visibly without disability—and thin? When any body that is even slightly larger than the mythical, impossible mean of television is obviously presented as locked into diet culture? Is it surprising that there is an epidemic of eating distress when we are presented with such an impossible version of "reality"? Silly TV may seem innocent, the least guilty of our pleasures (especially compared with reality TV, taken up below) but the impact of the few stories we're told, over and over again, gives us a pathway for a "correct" reality that can be very hard to escape.

REALITY TV

"Unscripted" or reality TV burst into ascendancy about 25 years ago, initially with shows like *Survivor* and *The Apprentice* alongside networks like TLC that aimed to showcase "real" life. Unscripted television now comprises a huge percentage of network offerings and the omnipresence of competitions, home renovations, makeovers and possible cakes—or not cakes—is overwhelming.

There are many tropes which recur across unscripted television, but two stand out in particular in regard to fat. The first is that much reality television is aspirational: the overwhelming number of real estate/renovation and other makeover offerings show viewers how to demand and create the life you want, in your environment and in your own body. These shows suggest that a better life is within our grasp and that, indeed, to refuse to actively participate in creating that life is a breach of the neoliberal contract.

In case we're confused about what happens if we're complacent about our lives or willing to just let things go, there is a whole other trope—the cautionary tale—waiting for us. Shows such as *The Biggest Loser* and a raft of other less successful weight loss shows not only position weight loss as possible and vitally necessary, but they also position participants as always having a sad back story, a reason why weight has arrived that is rooted in tragedy. Even shows such as *My Fat Fabulous Life*, which submits a medical reason for fat and aims to show the need for compassion toward fat people, nonetheless frames fat as tragic.

In its own particular category is the world of super-sized freak show reality TV. *My 600 Pound Life* followed on a series of "specials" (*Half Ton Man* and *The 750lb Man* for example) that are eerily similar to the fat lady at the carnival of old. We are invited to gawk at super sized people, to see them as inherently abject and impossible, unable to even wear clothes or walk, degrading both disability and fat in one fell swoop. The series opens with a disclaimer: "Each year, hundreds of weight loss operations are performed on patients weighting 600 pounds. Their chances of long-term success are less than five percent." This disclaimer would seem to suggest that fat is immutable and weight loss nearly impossible, but—through the use of humiliating images of naked supersized people being bathed and rolled over and otherwise framed in debased ways—quickly reminds us that even though most people will fail at losing weight, it is nonetheless incumbent upon everyone to try. It is not only the spectre of imminent death that is offered in these cases but also the impossibility of a livable life. Like all popular culture offerings, however, the show itself contributes to the view of very fat life as intrinsically horrible.

On her blog *The Fat Lip*, fat activist Ash writes the following about *My 600 Pound Life*:

> But the reality—and truly the cruelty—of this whole production is that it is designed to be a spectacle. The producers and doctors tell you, the 600 pound person being recruited by Gabe the casting assistant, that if you don't commit yourself to this "journey" and ultimately undergo this surgery, that you will die. Unequivocally. This is your only option to stay alive. But you are in luck! This show can save you! Only one tiny catch, though. Very minor. In order for the show to provide this *life-saving* (they INSIST it is life-saving) service, you must reveal your most vulnerable moments—your greatest emotional and physical struggles—to a national audience.
>
> Every fear and insecurity must be recorded. Every swollen limb gets a close-up. Have to step sideways through a doorway? Get that on camera. And boy are they ever going to need to film you eating. The producers of this show will take great care to show the parts of you that the audience will find most horrifying. They want you to seem grotesque. Monstrous. It is very important that your very existence seems as shocking and tragic as possible and that your body seems hideously inhuman.

But you must subject yourself to this—to being made a gruesome spectacle and cautionary tale—to *live*. These compassionate heroes will save your *life* for the low, low price of your actual human dignity.

(Ash 2020)

Importantly, Ash notes that the inability of fat activist spaces to absorb the experiences of superfat or infinifat people contributes to the desperation upon which the show capitalizes. She names the ways that people at the largest end of the spectrum are abandoned even by systems such as fat activism and Fat Studies. Ash reminds us that fat hatred does not start or end with popular media but also that its role can't be underestimated.

OTHER SITES

Of course, popular media is not restricted to literature, film and television. Love songs maintain a heterosexual and fairy-talesque bias. Professional sports are sexist and masculinist in their approach. Even if we never read a book or watch a movie or TV, we will still be made aware at every turn of how urgently we need to change our bodies.

As I write this, the Paris Olympics are in full swing, replete with endless ads for Ozempic. Olympic athletes are not "normal"—they are even more extreme physical outliers than those profiled on *My 600 Pound Life*—but we are nonetheless meant to view them as aspirational and inspiring—get off the couch and join them in the quest for personal betterment!

How many messages do you get about bodies and thinness? On any given day, try to catalogue how many different places you are given information about fatness and thinness. Are you exposed to advertisements on your daily commute? Does your employer want you to join their Weight Watchers group? Did your colleague comment on their indulgence over the weekend? Did your mom tell you to eat only half of whatever you were served? The ubiquity of messaging has become background noise such that it can be easy for all those messages to escape our notice. The result, however, of this relentless bombardment is that we continuously maintain our awareness of what a correct body should look like and how it should act. This impact is exhausting and overwhelming.

Every year, *People* magazine presents an issue about people who are now "Half Their Size!" Shrinking the body in half is meant to be inspiring and to motivate us to do the same. This issue is full of the same themes as reality TV—trite information on how success is achieved, blended with tragic back stories of why people "let themselves go" in the first place. Of course *People* magazine, even beyond these special issues, is part of the reason we are so mired in fatphobia—a periodical that claims to show "People" instead shows us an airbrushed, whitened, and absurdly thin version of who the "people" are. Aliens sent to this planet and prepared with *People* magazine would be greatly confused at the bodies of actual human beings. The messaging throughout all forms of media is the same— birth, adversity, triumph, success. When can we just rest?

Oprah Winfrey is arguably one of the most powerful women on the planet. She was, for many years, the world's only Black billionaire; her talk show ran for more than 25 years; she is viewed as one of the most influential people in the world (Wikipedia, "Oprah Winfrey" n.d.). She is, in some ways, the canonical story of the American Dream—triumphing over true adversity in her childhood, overcoming endless barriers and now universally recognized and beloved. For many years, Oprah Winfrey has had virtually every possible resource at her disposal—money, people, medicine. Yet the perennial story that has dogged her every accomplishment has been about her weight. Oprah Winfrey has been every possible size, has tried every possible intervention and has never stayed consistently thin. In 2015 she invested in Weight Watcher's rebranding, replete with marketing toward 8-year-olds (National Eating Disorders Association n.d.; Yang 2022); in 2024 she left the board of Weight Watchers because she is taking weight loss medication (instead?). **If Oprah Winfrey cannot lose weight, what hope is there for anyone else?** I understand that had she been consistently fat earlier in her career, she likely would not have achieved the success she has had, but what message would it send for her to just be happily fat now, to declare a truce in the war against her body?

SOCIAL MEDIA

I am middle-aged and as a result much of the media which informed my childhood was through film, television and commercials, as well as the books I endlessly read. My children, however, are living in an entirely different world. Social media is the predominant space in which most of us now learn about ourselves in the world: endless information offered in infinite tiny bites.

Social media and digital technologies are an incredibly influential part of popular culture. Our ability to engage with one another across huge distances in real time has made the world smaller—the infinitude of information has perhaps made it feel larger and more overwhelming. We can connect with friends and family and also consume content made by people who do not have traditional influence or access to sites of power. For the most part we are all equally able to view someone squishing some slime or watch a dog fall off a step.

In some respects we are living through a digital and technological revolution. Our constant access to curated information is unprecedented. Even 20 years ago the thought of most of the people on earth having access to mobile super computers would have been laughable. I don't mean to underestimate the digital divide—access to online technologies is not equally distributed and issues of age, education, poverty and geography do leave many people unable to access the digital world. That said, the ubiquity of cheap cell phone technologies has begun to shift the digital divide and mobile access is becoming more and more reachable across the globe.

While we communicate and consume media differently than we used to, all new forms of communication tend to preserve and reflect existing social mores. In other words: new technologies don't entirely predict new ways of thinking. Digital media reflects the same normativity of other media, showcasing whiteness and heterosexuality, avoiding disability and entrenching ideas about thinness. There is a deluge of new messages, but in many respects they maintain the same ideas we've always had. This is unsurprising, because we are mostly the same people making those messages—if we live in a culture that sees weight loss as obligatory and celebrates thinness, is it any surprise that 30% of the ads on my Instagram are for exercise/lifestyle/eating systems? Given our focus on celebrity and idealized visuality, isn't the use of filters and beautiful airbrushed lives just an obvious extension of our existing value system?

That said, the omnipresence of social media and digital technologies can be very overwhelming. The endless parade of "corrected" perfect bodies and lives can make it hard to remember what real flesh and body life looks like or feels like, and as such, social media can contribute to our epidemic of self-hatred and self-regulation. If we all want to look like the people on our phones—but even those people don't actually look like those people—how do we live with ourselves?

There is an abundance of curated and edited living happening online. Perfect motherhood, perfect charcuterie board, perfect garden, faultless soufflé, impeccable pores. Especially since the social isolation of COVID when so much of our connection was happening over screens, it is easy to forget that our bodies still poop and pee, that our skin can stretch, that our stains and scars can't simply be erased.

At the same time that social media merely reflects the deep normativity of our societies, there are new possibilities in digital space that are quite different than our pre-networked lives. Parents of children with unique diagnoses can find one another across space and time. Left-handed train nerds can form a Discord. And the fatties can begin to unpack the stories being told about them from all around the globe. Fat activism has existed for as long as there have been fat people, but the increasing speed with which we can connect across geography has made the possibility of fat connection greater and more robust. The suspicion we may feel—maybe my body *isn't* the problem?—can take root in community and connection in meaningful and important ways. We can seek out people like us, and we can also find images of bodies like ours, as an antidote to the relentless normativity with which we are surrounded.

How did you find this book? Were you googling "Fat Studies"? The ability for Fat Studies to take root beyond a few gender studies classrooms is partially due to the capacity for digital media to allow ideas to spread and flow.

Fat activist and author Lindy West responds to questions about her confidence by naming online culture:

> Honestly, this 'Where do you get your confidence?' chapter could be 16 words long. Because there was really only one step to my body acceptance: look at pictures of fat women on the internet until they don't make you uncomfortable any more. That was the entire process.
>
> (2016, 69)

The remedy for shame is so often pride and connection. Finding people who are like you, amplifying your voice in chorus, can be a way to reject the stories told about you and about bodies like yours. This is true for queer folks, contributes to anti-racist organizing, builds connection among neurodivergent people. It is especially true for fat people who may grow up steeped in shame and rejection and who can benefit so greatly from finding their people.

For example, Kotow considers the ways that online connection can mitigate social rejection. She writes that, "Finding online fat community that taught me I could learn to simply accept—and maybe even love—my fat body was a defining point in my life" (Kotow 2024, 181). Kotow explains that finding validation online allowed her the confidence to enter into real life fat spaces and consider that she would find community and solace there.

When humans began to communicate by telephone, naysayers were sure that the capacity for human conversation without embodied connection signalled the end of civilization. Each time we have changed how we communicate we have changed human connections in important ways. On the whole, we have maintained the same mores, strengths and faults we already have, but each change in communication technology has also opened new opportunities. Fat people do not have easier lives because of the internet and social media; they do not have worse lives because of them, either. Rather, fat life has changed and morphed as a result of the changes around us, and will continue to change as these systems evolve further.

FASHION

Clothes are interesting because they matter across the whole hierarchy of needs. At their most basic, clothes keep us protected from the weather and maintain a level of privacy. At the highest levels of fashion, clothes may function as artistry, self-expression, political messaging or otherwise in aid of personal fulfilment. In the grand scheme of ways that fat people are limited and put down by the world, clothing may seem like an incidental concern, but given the impact of clothing on how we understand ourselves and how we are understood by those around us, fashion is a meaningful part of popular culture and fat people's inability to fully partake in this function of fashion is problematic and painful.

While fat is a fluid signifier and attempts to demarcate "stages" of fat can be problematic, there are specific experiences of fat and of fat phobia that shift across the size spectrum. These experiences are particularly delineated in thinking through issues of access to clothing. Ashley of The Fat Lip podcast offers a gentle categorization scheme as a way of thinking through the impacts of fatphobia, in regard to clothing and beyond, for people of different sizes.

Ash describes "The Fat Spectrum, as used on www.thefatlip.com" and presents four options: The first says "Small Fat: 1x–2x, 18 and lower, Torrid 00 to 1: Find clothes that fit at mainstream brands and can shop in many stores". The second says "Mid Fat: 2x–3x, 20–24, Torrid 2 or 3. Shop at some mainstream brands, but mostly dedicated plus brands and online". The third says "Superfat: 4x–5x, 26–32, Torrid 4 to 6. Wear the highest sizes at plus brands. Can often only shop online". The final description says "Infinifat: 6x and higher, 34 and higher, some Torrid 6. Very difficult to find anything that fits, even online. Often requires custom sizing".

It is virtually impossible to engage in human society without some kind of access to clothing. Before any considerations of red carpet chic, we must simply cover our bodies and even staples like underwear can be difficult to find at the largest end of the spectrum. I think about a research participant I encountered via one of my graduate students who, in order to wear underpants, had to sew together the backsides of two pairs of mid-fat undies to make one functional pair for her shape and size.

I often think of privilege vs. oppression in terms of mental load. The privilege to simply replace underpants as needed is available to some people: poverty, ability, as well as fat, may limit this capacity. The added step of needing to MacGyver together underpants simply to have something to wear is not something that occurs to the vast majority of people.

As articulated by the chart above, the bigger you get, the more you fall off the hierarchy of needs. Smaller fat people may be able to indulge in self-expression, albeit to a lesser extent than thinner people; larger fat people may struggle to simply cover themselves in any way. Further, there is a flattening of style occurring: One of the impacts of colonization is that access to purpose-made community clothing is continuously diminishing, replaced by mass market fast fashion. In other words: we all need to get dressed and the expectation is increasingly that we can wear the same jeans and hoodies as one another no matter where we are and what we look like.

All of these issues matter. By acknowledging differential access to clothing across the fat spectrum I don't aim to hierarchize fat experiences—instead, I would like to suggest that access to clothing that covers our bodies *and* makes us feel authentically good should be a baseline for all bodies. Calla Evans' work acknowledges that there are so few dresses available in 5x and 6x that people routinely show up to the event wearing the same clothes (2020, 20). While potentially a bonding experience, it is also painful to be unable to access the full palette of human expression through dress. Fat is not the only reason people's choices are limited, but it is one that matters.

These issues may be even more acute in the intersections of experience and identity. Fat non-binary folks may struggle to emulate an androgynous aesthetic that seems to revolve around bony leanness. Sonia Meerai acknowledges the particular pain that comes in trying to buy a wedding sari and hearing the "riiiiip" as the largest size fails to accommodate her body (2020). Fundamentally, we do not only want that jeans and hoodie—we may want flamboyance or conservatism, severe tailoring or ruffles galore. We may want to wear a kurta or an abeya or a bikini or a football jersey or all of these at the same time. We are not singularities, and our fat bodies do not foreclose the rest of our identities, so the narrowing of our options to the skulls-and-Hello-Kitty style of Torrid (for those of us lucky enough to fit!) does not allow the full range of human experience.

FATSHION

Partially aided by the rise of social media, fat people have become increasingly able to share fashion hacks and images of themselves in outfits of the day. Some of these outfits are cobbled together through self-made garments and vintage finds while others are off-the-rack (or off-the-website) finds. While the burgeoning interest in fat fashion represents a meaningful site of fat resistance, it is still largely limited to people in the small and mid-fat range of the fat spectrum—indeed, precisely as more mainstream retailers respond to demands for diversity by stretching their clothes into 1x–3x fits, people 4x and above are left in the dust with fewer and fewer options. And as Ash writes—what of the folks who live where sizes end? Ash notes:

> But what should we fats on the very very very fat end of the fat spectrum be called? I humbly propose "infinifat". Because what size am I? I really have no fucking idea. A size greater than any assignable size number. Infinity?
>
> (cited in Evans 2020, 5)

The revolutionary potential of fat activism in popular culture will be explored below, and fatshion is undoubtedly a big part of that reclamation. Ash's words, however, should be a sobering reflection on the limits of who can reclaim space.

RESISTANCE IN POPULAR CULTURE

Reading this chapter, it can be tempting to believe that fat people are doomed: at worst bullied and at best ignored in popular culture. That said, while there is an overwhelming array of fatphobic and fat hating media, popular culture is also a meaningful site of resistance.

Beginning in the realm of literature, there is a tiny but growing field of children's picture books that take up body acceptance. Books like *Beautifully Me* and *Bodies Are Cool* do not explicitly position fat bodies but begin from a notion of bodies as variable and diverse. *Abigail and the Whale* stands out as a rare children's storybook that centres fat from a positive orientation.

Moving into chapter books, *Starfish* by Lisa Fipps does not shy away from acknowledging fat phobia and presents a protagonist who speaks back and takes up space. There are a range of young adult books, some of which are anthologies of first person experiences and others which are fiction. Julie Murphy's offerings, including *Dumplin'* and *Pudding*, as well as the superhero graphic novel *Faith Taking Flight* stand out in this field but more can be explored here: https://www.epicreads.com/blog/fat-protagonists/.

For adults, there has been an array of memoirs that explore fat life from a range of positionalities. *Shrill* by Lindy West, Roxane Gay's *Hunger, Heavy* by Kiese Laymon and *Thick* by Tressie McMillan Cottam are all excellent reads that speak back to the usual story of fat; the latter three books also explicitly name the impacts of fat Black life in America. There is also a growing field of thicker protagonists in romance novels and "women's" literature such as Jennifer Weiner and Talia Hibbert's books. The appetite for these books is becoming more evident and as a result, authors that centre fat characters are more likely to reach the market.

In the realm of mainstream films, there are spinoffs of some of the books listed above, notably *Dumplin'*. That said, the majority of fat friendly movies are documentaries such as *Fattitude* (2017) or the 2023 film *Your Fat Friend* which profiles fat activist and author Aubrey Gordon. Similarly, in the realm of television there are several televised series that are based on fat activist memoirs, notably *Shrill* in the US and *My Mad, Fat Diary* in the UK. Somehow, first person experience allows for fat friendly fiction in a way that creative storytelling still limits. In the realm of reality TV, while *My Fat Fabulous Life* is still somewhat problematic, it is nonetheless the story of a largely happy superfat person and as such is still a radical offering. Other shows that are meant to objectify and humiliate fat people such as *Here Comes Honey Boo Boo* may nonetheless lend themselves to a more radical read by showcasing unashamed fat people (Friedman 2014).

Perhaps unsurprisingly, however, the mainstream mechanisms of publishing, filmmaking and the television industry are slow to adopt fat friendly stories. Further, mainstream media seems to only allow one standard deviation from the mythical norm—you can be fat as long as you're white, queer as long as you're not disabled, etc. For most people, life is isn't regimented into fragments this way, and the specifics of our lived experience may require an awareness of diversity that is missing even from—perhaps especially from—media that explores fat life. For this and many other reasons, much of the positive representation of fat life and capacity for fat community begins through the internet.

So much of the resistance—like so much of the hatred—occurs online. The ease of storytelling in social media settings, YouTube channels and other online sites allows for a virtually instantaneous platform for self-discovery. Social media can condemn fat people savagely, but it can also inspire alternative tellings of fat, which can assist in the spreading of fat solidarity and activism. Over the years I've heard from many students and other young people about how the first interruption to the diet narrative of fat life came through social media and felt literally life-saving. Through sharing hacks for how to move fat bodies through space (and in airplanes), learning more about how to creatively clothe ourselves, into the realm of fat friendly family planning and fertility advice, the networked world has offered a wealth of knowledge and connection to many different disenfranchised people, including fat folks.

The internet allows us to find people who are living specifically like us, rather than offering generalizations—I can find other fat social work academics thinking about fat activism in the human services; I can find fat students navigating campus life; fat weight lifting or rock climbing communities abound—I can find friends, sex, cooking tips, chess clubs, advice on the right bicycle, awareness of my experience with fat and disability. While the fat activist world is still pitched toward whiteness, the level of diversity and variegation is better online than elsewhere, and as more and more folks participate, we create a multicoloured, diverse and truly complicated world that better showcases our experiences and desires.

Fat people are, generally, unseen and misunderstood. Yet there is room for hope here, in considering the ways that fat voices are finally being heard, albeit in the corners. For now, especially in mainstream media spaces, fat people are seldom presented positively, and the rare positive story centres fat experience as the key issue—fat people are still remarkable, even when shown with care. The hope is that there will be such a range of fat experiences and stories that fatness will become unremarkable, just another possible way of being human in the world.

MOVING ON

Popular culture is like a fun house mirror—it reflects back our belief systems, biases and values, but equally, impacts how we think and live. Popular culture, including digital media and social networks, has a huge impact on how we understand the value of specific bodies in the world; yet someone had to have these ideas in order for them to proliferate in the first place. Changing the stories we tell is therefore slow and iterative, shifting our collective public understanding of who matters and why. While the proliferation of alternative fat stories is beginning to take hold, these stories are still woefully under-diversified. Fat Studies and fat activism have rightly been accused of being white woman's fields describing white women's problems. Yet fat people exist in every possible range of human experience. Furthermore, the specifics of fatphobia, racism and colonization have an especially pernicious impact on fat racialized and Indigenous people.

The next chapter will begin to explore some of the specific impacts of fat in conjunction with other lived experiences. While acknowledging that all identity categories may flatten difference and hierarchize humanity, it is important nonetheless to explore some of the specific impacts of fat life alongside experiences of racism or marginalized gender identity or sexual orientation; in relation to experiences of disability; and alongside other circumscribed experiences such as motherhood.

FURTHER READING

Abdillahi, Idil and Friedman, May. "Lessons Learned from Fat Women on Television." *Body Stories: In and out and With and Through Fat*, edited by Jill Andrew and May Friedman, Demeter Press, 2020, pp. 165–172.

Barry, Ben. "Fabulous Masculinities: Refashioning the Fat and Disabled Male Body." *Fashion Theory: The Journal of Dress, Body and Culture*, vol. 23, no. 2, 2019, pp. 275–307.

Cleary, Krystal. "Misfitting and Hater Blocking: A Feminist Disability Analysis of the Extraordinary Body on Reality Television." *Disability Studies Quarterly*, vol. 36, no. 4, 2016, pp. 61–66.

Hass, Margaret. After the After: The Biggest Loser and Post-Makeover Narrative Trajectories in Digital Media. *Fat Studies*, vol. 6, no. 2, 2016, pp. 135–151.

WORKS CITED

"17 YA Books Featuring Fat, Female Protagonists." *Epic Reads*. https://www. epicreads.com/blog/fat-protagonists/. Accessed October 1, 2024.

Ash. "Our 600 Pound Lives." *The Fat Lip*. http://thefatlip.com/2020/03/21/ our-600-pound-lives/. Accessed July 22, 2024.

Bruusgaard, Emily. "'I'd Wish to Be Tall and Slender': L. M. Montgomery's Anne Series and the Regulatory Role of Slimness." *Fat Studies in Canada: Re(Mapping) the Field*, edited by Allison Taylor, Kelsey Ioannoni, Ramanpreet Annie Bahra, Calla Evans, Amanda Striver and May Friedman, Inanna Press, 2023, pp. 204–220.

Cali, Davide and Sonia Bougaeva. *Abigail and the Whale*, Owlkids, 2016.

Evans, Calla. "You Aren't What You Wear: An Exploration into Infinifat Identity Construction and Performance through Fashion." *Fashion Studies*, vol. 3, no. 1, 2020, pp. 1–31.

Feder, Tyler. *Bodies Are Cool*, Rocky Pond Books, 2021.

Fipps, Lisa. *Starfish*, Nancy Paulsen Books, 2021.

Friedman, May. "Here Comes a Lot of Judgment: Honey Boo Boo as a Site of Reclamation and Resistance." *Journal of Popular Television*, vol. 2, no. 1, 2014, pp. 77–95.

Gay, Roxane. *Hunger: A Memoir of (My) Body*, HarperCollins, 2017.

Kent, Clarkisha. "'Fat Monica' Is the Ghost That Continues to Haunt *Friends* 25 Years Later." *Entertainment Weekly*, September 4, 2019. https://ew. com/tv/2019/09/04/fat-monica-friends-25-years-later/.

Laymon, Kiese. *Heavy: An American Memoir*, Thorndike Press, 2019.

Lind, Emily R. M. "Queering Fat Activism: A Study in Whiteness." *Thickening Fat: Fat Bodies, Intersectionality and Social Justice*, edited by May Friedman, Carla Rice and Jen Rinaldi, Routledge, 2020, pp. 183–194.

McMillan Cottom, Tressie. *Thick: And Other Essays*, New Press, 2019.

Meerai, Sonia. "Taking Up Space in the Doctor's Office: How My Racialized Fat Body Confronts Medical Discourse." *Thickening Fat: Fat Bodies, Intersectionality and Social Justice*, edited by May Friedman, Carla Rice and Jen Rinaldi, Routledge, 2020, pp. 90–96.

My 600 Pound Life. TV show. TLC Network. 2012–present.

National Eating Disorders Association. "NEDA Statement on Kurbo by WW App." n.d. https://www.nationaleatingdisorders.org/neda-statem ent-kurbo-ww-app/. Accessed October 4, 2024.

Noor, Nabela. *Beautifully Me*, Simon and Schuster, 2021.

"Oprah Winfrey". *Wikipedia*, Wikimedia Foundation. https://en.wikipedia. org/wiki/Oprah_Winfrey. Accessed October 4, 2024.

West, Lindy. *Shrill: Notes from a Loud Woman*, Hachette Books, 2016.

Yang, Maya. "Weight Watchers Allegedly Used Diet App to Illegally Gather Data on Children, FTC Says." *The Guardian*, March 4, 2022. https://www.theguardian.com/society/2022/mar/04/weight-watchers-kurbo-diet-app-children-data Accessed October 2, 2024.

6

INTERSECTING FAT

INTRODUCTION

While fat stigma occurs to all kinds of people, both Fat Studies and much fat activism can tend to focus more on fat white women. Although intersectionality is threaded throughout this book with many different examples, this chapter seeks to look at some of the specific ways that fat intersects and interlocks with other lived experiences and identities. The chapter will look at some of the academic work that has contributed to Fat Studies as like other experiences (i.e. drawing from disability studies) or with other experiences (i.e. fatphobia as anti-Black racism). In offering a "thicker" view of fat, this chapter considers some of the areas of further thinking and research that may be required.

This chapter is framed by the following questions:

- How does fat life specifically and particularly impact Black, Indigenous and people of colour, people with different gender and sexualities, and people with different abilities?
- What is the impact of fat on parenthood and family structure?
- Where are different social struggles aligned with fat justice and where do they diverge?

Fat Studies is a young field and it is continuously being revised. Generic responses to fat life have tended to flatten difference and focus on normative experiences of race, class, ability, gender and beyond. This chapter seeks to explore some of the specific ways that fat impacts lives in the intersections as well as the ways that Fat Studies has begun to interrupt this limitation.

DOI: 10.4324/9781003539773-6

This is tricky work—organizing the world into specific categories and fixed markings is somewhat contrary to the spirit of Fat Studies, which aims to explore the messiness of life and to explode static categories. Any exploration of fat and disabled life, for example, will fall woefully short of a true consideration of all the intricacies that people may experience, based on specific disabilities, visible vs. invisible experiences, small or supersized fat life, and so on and so on. It is tempting to continue to just talk about fat people broadly and to avoid the pitfalls of focusing on specific identities, knowing how limiting such an analysis can be. That said: the specifics matter, and without choosing to deliberately centre specific experiences we tend to default toward normativity. This chapter is not capable of providing an exhaustive account of the many different intersectional fat experiences humans live through, but begins to provide a high level overview of the ways that fat life is experienced in relation to other identity categories with their own struggles and marginalizations.

OVERVIEW

Perhaps it is unsurprising, given the weight of evidence of how reviled fat people are, that when fat people are living in other marginalized identities, there are specific permutations of fat hatred which emerge. This is not math, and I reject the framing of intersectionality that is positioned as a recipe with different ingredients. We all dip in and out of different identifiable and hard-to-explain experiences, some of which may fit neatly into specific categories and some which may not; even among "named" categories, however, there is an infinite diversity of experience. Eli Clare writes,

> How do we make the space to talk honestly and wrenchingly about all the multi-layered systems of injustice that target some of us and privilege others for who we are? The layers are so tangled: gender folds into disability, disability wraps around class, class strains against race, race snarls into sexuality, sexuality hangs onto gender, all of it finally piling into our bodies.

(2003, p. 1)

Fat, too, is wildly diverse in its manifestations and experiences, based on size, context and myriad other possibilities. *Lives vary.* Given this clunky disclaimer, however, it is impossible to proceed without acknowledging that, for a lot of fat people of colour, tropes about laziness and productivity may fold over race and through fat, resulting in difficulty in figuring out where racism begins and fatphobia takes over. People with chronic health conditions or illnesses that require medical specialists may have a unique experience of fat and fatphobia based on the intricacies of their health status. There are high level working truths we must absorb here while also acknowledging the complexity and diversity of our experiences.

Further, we must acknowledge that our experiences are dynamic and variable: what is racist at work might be banter at home or in community; our bodies may be celebrated in our bedrooms but still rejected by our doctors; what is hot when we're 20 may be abhorrent when we're 60. Moving through time changes our bodies and the reactions to them; moving through space likewise has impacts on our fat lives but also our variable intersections. Many of us from immigrant and refugee families have had the experience of moving, almost instantaneously, from being the "usual" type of person, to being emphatically Other.

Given the chaos caused by space, time and differences among us, is it productive to explore specific identity categories? We must acknowledge that in doing so, we will narrow difference. We will get things wrong, gather the wrong people in, leave some people out. Yet to turn away from difference for fear of this flattening allows the invisible norms to be maintained. In the realm of fat life, this means centring the experiences of young, white, mid-fat women to the exclusion of others. With all this in mind: let us dive in.

RACE

As Sabrina Strings and DaShaun Harrison display, the origins of fatphobia are inescapably woven through the origins of racism, and especially anti-Black racism. The nation building project that reified self-improvement and a specific physique to follow was rooted in the degradation and theft of Black people following the Middle Passage and has been maintained through tropes of both Blackness and fatness that see specific bodies as less than human. Similarly, colonization framed Indigenous peoples as savage and saw the plunder of both people and land as a justifiable form of greed. Fatphobia is a shapeshifter, not held to any consistent logic. The pernicious stereotypes and abuses aimed at Black, Indigenous and other people of colour thus get re-purposed for fat people as evidence of a lack of humanity.

Given these historical roots, and the contemporary focus on fat communities of colour as particularly in need of intervention, it is therefore frustrating to have Fat Studies and fat activism characterized as not relevant to people of colour.

There are two main ways that this critique gets framed: first, that many different racialized communities celebrate bigger sizes and as such, are not harmed by eating distress or diet culture to the same extent as white folks. The second, is that in the face of rampant and extreme racism, fatphobia is an indulgence for which we cannot spare activist energy. Neither of these frameworks withstand scrutiny.

Community mores around size are quite variable across difference. What is "too fat" in one culture or community might be seen as scrawny elsewhere. I vividly remember a friend who was met by his grandma, back home, with the phrase "look at you, so nice and fat!" offered as a compliment. (I also remember all of us as teenagers, giggling at the idea that this could *ever* be framed as a positive statement, and my friend, like me, a culture-crossing child of immigrants, struggling with the competing messaging of his granny's statement.)

Tressie Cottom McMillan writes about learning about the different frames of attractiveness while watching the movie *Grease* in middle school and the moment where a white classmate was clearly mesmerized by Olivia Newton-John in leather pants in the final scenes of the movie:

I remember the scene so clearly because that was when I got it. A whole other culture of desirability had been playing out just above and beyond my awareness, while my mostly black and Latino friends traded jokes at gapped thighs, flat behinds, and never trusting a big butt and a smile. And when the teacher, a

> middle-aged white woman not unlike the one who once told me
> my breasts were too distracting, looked at the too-tall boy, she
> smiled at him and rolled her eyes, acknowledging his sexual
> appreciation of Sandy as normal if unmannerly. He smiled back
> and kind of shrugged as if to say, "I just can't help myself." The
> teacher and the too-tall boy were in cahoots. Sandy, that strange
> creature, was beautiful.
>
> (2019, 43)

I have yet to learn of a community that doesn't uphold some metric of desirability, so while many different communities "allow" for a range of embodiments that vary from the blond Barbie version of the norm, they may still have a norm, and may police one another within these normative expectations. Perhaps more importantly, people of colour still live within the larger world and as such, even if they live in bodies that are framed as desirable in home spaces, they may still face specific intersectional forms of fatphobia beyond their families and communities. In other words: you may think it's weird that Sandy is beautiful, but you still need to exist in a world in which she is the ideal to which you must aspire.

Other intersections yield other permutations and challenges. Fat Studies scholar Sucharita Sarkar explores the ways that the "yummy mummy" trope has entered into Indian culture, with Indian mothers facing dual competing expectations: to nourish their children endlessly, per Indian traditions, and simultaneously to worship thinness and Western beauty standards, for both mothers and their children (2020). Sarkar's work speaks to the perniciousness of thinness as a colonizing force that has spread throughout the globe as a by-product of Western belief systems. Boero finds similar outcomes in considering fat Latinx parents and kids in the spaces of child welfare—tropes of "good" parenting are overlaid with stories of size and race in order to demonize and chastise people of colour (2009).

Sanders explores the ways that discourses of obesity epidemic have been deployed to uphold whiteness and police race, and explicitly considers the feminization of fatness and the ways that Black fat women get framed (2019). The demonization of Black people and other racialized folks who are fat is increasing. Dorothy

Roberts speaks to the preponderance of "race-based medicine" that would seem to meet the unique needs of people of colour but are instead often simply money-grabs for pharmaceutical companies that maintain stories of non-white bodies as inferior and flawed (2010). Many of the conditions being targeted may co-exist with fat. In the present day context where there is concern about behaviour being deemed racist, fatphobic interventions may allow for racist hatred to proliferate without being stopped.

Anna Mollow specifically explores the ways that fat Black bodies are deemed "unvictimizable" in the context of police violence and beyond (2017). She names the ways that larger Black bodies, especially those of men, are viewed as terrifying and dangerous; but notes that simultaneously, when Black people such as Eric Garner are harmed, their intrinsic ill health must be to blame:

> defenders of the officers who killed Garner reproduced stereotypes of black bodies as inherently disabled when they insisted that fatness-induced disabilities—rather than a deadly police chokehold—caused Garner's death. At the same time, Garner was portrayed as almost superhumanly invulnerable when Congressman King described him as a "350-pound person who was resisting arrest," the implication being that Garner's size made him so dangerous that deadly force was necessary to defuse the threat that he presented .... fatphobia and ableism work in conjunction with racism to construct an ideological double bind that rhetorically positions black bodies as incapable of being victimized. One side of this double bind renders violence against black people inconsequential by suggesting that fatness is the real cause of any injuries inflicted upon them, while its other side depicts violence as a necessary response to the excessive physical power that black people, especially those who are fat, are imagined to embody.
>
> (Mollow 2017, 105)

Mollow explores the ways that fat Black bodies are viewed as defective, considering the ways that economic and ecological racism have impacted communities of colour that are then held accountable for shifts in health outcomes.

Health is the new wealth. While poverty was historically seen as due to personal failings and thus was a valid reason to police—literally and figuratively—people of colour, discourses of health are increasingly the currency for abuse of people on the basis of race, ethnicity and migration. Fears about unfit immigrants are pervasive throughout the history of settler colonial nations such as the US and Canada, but the specific nuances of fears about excess spending based on obesity-related health conditions—many of which are strongly correlated with the stress responses many migrant people experience because of the challenges of coming to a new place—result in the specific disciplining of certain bodies under the guise of health but through age-old racist logics. The perniciousness of fears about fat are thus a major tool in the arsenal of health witch hunts that can be deliberately and effectively deployed toward people of colour. The social determinants of health are less likely to be achievable because of conditions of racism, and yet less likely to be possible for fat people: fat people of colour are thus more likely to experience health distress but especially likely to be found responsible for their own challenges.

INDIGENEITY AND COLONIZATION

For the First Peoples of settler colonial states, there have been endless grave injustices. Beginning with the notion of the land as empty, ignoring its inhabitants, the land and its people continue to be pillaged and abused. Residential schools, mass graves, missing Indigenous women and girls, the lack of clean water—it is impossible to catalogue the injustices that Indigenous people have faced and continue to face. Further, given the deep connection to the land, the ecological injustices that are done in the name of "progress" further inflict damage on Indigenous people and communities, both practically and psychically. At the same time, the story of Indigeneity isn't a story of victimhood, a tale of abjection. There is enormous resilience and resurgence throughout groups of First Nations, Native, Inuit, Metis and other Indigenous groups.

Margaret Robinson details a range of ways in which the conquest of Indigenous peoples is linked to discourses about fat (2020).

She explores Western high art from the 16th century that portrays the pillaging of stolen land, with Indigenous bodies being framed as savage, voracious and also fat—the spoils of the land being plundered. Further, Robinson explores the ways that contemporary health funding in the Canadian context is deeply concerned with Indigenous health in the realm of obesity and diabetes prevention while being eerily silent about state failures to provide obvious social determinants of health such as clean water. Finally, Robinson's work undertakes a visual analysis of a Health Canada poster that shows a (seemingly) Indigenous family striving for health:

> The grandmother, in the centre background, stands at the counter touching green-topped carrots. In the left foreground, the mother chops celery at the kitchen table, smiling at her toddler who eats cut-up fruit from a white bowl. In the back right, the father stirs something at the stove. The eyeline of both parents is on the child, framing Indigenous parents as responsible for the size and health of their children.
>
> The kitchen reflects middle-class values of cleanliness and consumerism: the white gas stove has a digital readout; there is a white dishwasher; a white coffeemaker is nestled behind a bowl of fruit on the counter. All the objects in the room are new, and white dominates in cabinets, window frame, and blinds. The sparking silver faucet over the sink indicates this is not one of the many First Nations families living without running water.

(2020, 23)

Robinson's analysis shows the multi-pronged force of fatphobia as both an outpost of colonization as well as a tool in the arsenal of colonizing states. The focus on a specific Western view of "progress" and success, the emphasis on weights and measures and numeric frameworks—all lead to an inescapable fixation on fat. In the realm of Indigenous folks, the discourses of Native bodies as wrong has been threaded through the story of theft and annihilation. The present day health witch hunt that centres Indigenous bodies as inferior and prone to disease is simply a new retelling of the same story. Fundamentally this story inflates personal responsibility for health and prosperity while flattening any acknowledgment of the impact of colonization or the responsibility of governments and other structures for the people and lands from which everything was stolen.

Thinking through fat and colonization can also have another angle: The spread of Western cultural norms throughout the globe is happening at a dizzying pace, aided by popular culture and social media. There is almost no place on earth where you can't buy a Coke and, following this logic, almost nowhere that you can't buy a Diet Coke. Now: full disclosure, Diet Coke is my beloved beverage of choice—so refreshing and bubbly!—but the ubiquity of its spread and the semantic shift of the word "diet" as merely a benign descriptor, rather than evidence of a pernicious global discourse of weight loss as viable and necessary, should be alarming.

In "Fashion, its Sacrifice Zone, and Sustainability" Niessen (2020) details the shift away from artisanal and Indigenous forms of clothing creation toward instead the ubiquity of Western clothes. This is a sad shift for so many reasons—the loss of historic and generational skills, the move toward plastic based clothing that is a disaster for the planet—but it also speaks to an aesthetic flattening that ensures that all bodies are dressed similarly all over the globe, with traditional clothing being relegated to costume. Blue jeans are an especially interesting example: made of cotton and indigo that is often grown under inhumane and environmentally irresponsible conditions, increasingly threaded through with plastics and non-biodegradable components, jeans are both ubiquitous and dangerous. Not all bodies are designed for jeans; and jeans are not a neutral or innocent choice. Weather, size, ethnicity, genetics all speak to the need for a range of clothing choices, but these choices are being flattened as Western expectations and mores spread. Unfortunately, shifts in clothes result in changes in embodied expectations as well—while prior to the Industrial Revolution all clothes were made for the bodies of the wearer, now it is very hard to go anywhere where clothes are created with specific bodies and measurements in mind. As a result, the same sizes and silhouettes are increasingly venerated as a by-product of Western cultural drift. Fashion magazines may show models in a range of hues, but those models have eerily similar bodies. While this impact may not meet the official definition of colonization, it is a new form of meta-colonization that takes the diversity of culture worldwide and instead replaces it with Diet Cokes and jeans.

In the realm of food, things are also dire: traditional food choices are often sneered at by doctors and dieticians who operate from

Western and white information about diet and weight. As we have seen, however, these logics are not actually terribly well informed and they may simply serve as a way of imposing white Western logics over food choices. The Diet Coke is thus paired with a slice of pizza and a vegan bowl while the plethora of global food choices are repackaged for a Western palate at the Chinese buffet. I do not mean to suggest that there are "good" and "bad" foods—all food has a role, but food is also discursive and the narrowing of food choices has implications for the earth and its inhabitants. While approximately a quarter of the globe experiences food insecurity and risk of starvation, the popular story that proliferates is that an emaciated physique is attractive. The disconnect between people's lived realities and the cultural story of food, fat and bodies that is continuously spread around the globe is dismaying. Fat-phobia is a sharp tool in colonization's arsenal, but one that has become so normalized and invisibilized that its reach is barely acknowledged.

DISABILITY

There is both strong alliance and great unease in the blending of disability and fat activism. This may present specific challenges for people living in this intersection. Finding a fat friendly family doctor is challenging—finding a fat friendly oncologist or gastro-intestinal specialist may be even harder. A fat person with mobility challenges may face sneering rather than the unfortunate blend of compassion and pity faced by other mobility device users. Health conditions may cause fat but may inevitably be seen as being caused *by* fat—the usual fight to be taken seriously in healthcare settings is exacerbated in the case of fat life with disability. The theoretical work extends this challenge and meets it in a range of different ways.

There is significant scholarship exploring the relationship between fat and disability. In some work, fat is viewed as being like a disability—fat bodies are normal, but living in a world that is actively designed against them (Cooper, 2007) Other authors explore the ways that fat activism can and must align with disability justice in the quest for all bodies to be welcomed and respected (Herndon 2002; Meleo-Erwin 2014). Much of this research draws on the social model of disability which understands all impairment as stemming from hostile environments rather than bodies with different abilities.

One problem with the social model of disability is that it does not acknowledge that disability is not equally distributed. Mollow writes that "For many black people ... who face ongoing threats to their physical and mental health from racism, overwork, poverty, and lack of access to health care—a politics purporting not to care about health is not viable" (2017, 112). Acknowledging racial and environmental injustice and their differential impacts on different communities should not end with a degradation of disability as fundamentally flawed. How do we, for example, speak to the impacts of lead poisoning in poorer communities without suggesting that the different neurological and cognitive capacities of people with lead poisoning are evidence of less worthy lives? These are tangled questions, and fat justice lives in the middle of this snarl, considering why some bodies have greater access to health, wealth and safety and what happens to those who do not. This circles back to the notion of fat as choice—our differential access to privilege is another of many reasons why our bodies will be different. Mollow suggests the need for fat, Black disability studies as a form of activism:

> Fat black disability studies should take a multipronged approach that opposes the medical profession's equation of fatness with disease, underscores the value of ill and disabled people's lives, and at the same time resists the unfair distribution of health risks along lines of race, body size, and ability.
>
> (2017, 114)

While it is essential to acknowledge the embeddedness of racism and colonization as well as capitalism in creating different forms of access to health and ability, it is equally essential that the bodies we have now, in this world, are honoured and supported. A framework that connects fat rights to disability justice can draw on a bigger logic of embodied justice that includes many forms of non-normativity. There is a far greater range of possible bodies than the seats on public transportation or the makeup counter at the drugstore might suggest. By bringing fat justice and disability rights together under a bigger canopy of embodiment work there is room to include people who may move back and forth or between fat and disability at various points in their lives as well as leaving room for ambiguous embodiments that don't adhere to the logic of identities as concrete categories. With that being said: some fat people do not want to be associated with disability, seeing that frame as part of a story of fat bodies as inferior. Some disability activists do not want to extend justice to fat bodies, seeing these bodies as detracting from the bigger fight for inclusion by people with "real" struggles. These are uneasy bedfellows.

Drawing from this unease, there is a significant strand of fat activism that seeks to explore the ways that fat is *not* like disability, suggesting that fat people can be healthy and fit and that, in opposition to bodies with disability, fat bodies are not impaired. Much of this logic comes from frames such as Health At Every Size, explored in greater detail elsewhere. Obviously this logic is problematic in that it positions disability and ill health as inherently negative and thus seeks to distance fat people from these conditions and identities. In addition, this stance dismisses the existence of people who are both fat and living with disability or imperfect health—something that will be true of almost all people at some point.

Meleo-Erwin asks us to disrupt this logic, suggesting that normalizing fatness is a losing strategy that will ultimately pathologize most people and behaviours (2014). Instead, Meleo-Erwin recommends that we embrace "freakery" and lean into the non-normative as a celebrated and respected state, in and beyond fat. As can be seen in the analysis of popular media in Chapter 5, children learn about normalcy early and often, and there are high costs throughout the lifespan for deviating from the norm. Meleo-Erwin writes that "in contemporary Western societies people are primarily disciplined through and regulated through their active engagement with recommended practices and techniques designed to normalize their behaviour, selves and bodies" (2014, 391). Fat activist approaches that aim to fit into this framework are doomed to failure because most fat people will never be normal enough, but also because bodies are dynamic and even bodies that are "normal" will move farther and farther from this state throughout the lifespan. As a result, acknowledging that most of us are freaks—and that all of us are heading toward freakery—allows for a response to fat hatred that builds alliances, acknowledges our intersections and also is politically robust in its rejection of capitalist and colonialist logics.

GENDER

Fat lands differently based on gender, and fatphobia can also be deployed in distinct ways dependent on how a body is read across the gender spectrum. Expectations of male and female bodies, as well as bodies outside the binary, vary across a range of different intersections but are often quite distinct based on gender.

In "Is Fat a Feminist Issue? Exploring the Gendered Nature of Weight Bias", Fikkan and Rothblum explore the specific ways that fatphobia is an agent of sexism that can be used in specific and debilitating ways to demean women (2012). Certainly, the focus on attractiveness, dress and demure femininity is a big part of disciplining female bodies and ensuring that women are too preoccupied or demoralized to keep track of all the different axes of patriarchy. Diet culture largely hones in on female-identified people, and there is a case to be made that in most cultures the acceptable boundaries for a female body are narrower than those for men. While female fat has historically been associated with fertility, in the present moment fat women are targeted for fearmongering about infertility and cautioned of the harms they may cause their offspring should they manage to become pregnant.

Within dating and relationship spaces, fat women's value is limited. In heterosexual contexts, men who find fat women attractive are seen as perverts, as though an attraction to fat must always be evidence of fetish. The social currency afforded fat women is so low that any traditional form of progress or success—marriage, employment, education—is harder to achieve and may be met with surprise or dubiousness, especially for racialized fat women.

Men are not immune to the impacts of fatphobia. While men continue to be adjudicated more on performance than attractiveness, there is an increasing push toward mandatory attractiveness and grooming practices for men. The visual expectation of what an executive, or a doctor, or a professor looks like are different for men than women, and the in-built advantage of masculinity may still assist fat men more than women of any size, but increasingly there is a focus on sculpting, manscaping and other body management practices. Centuries of female anxiety about appearance have resulted in a very lucrative industry that is spreading to include men. As a result, diet culture and fat phobia—and a specific increase in health anxiety—has functioned to discipline men. The need to be strong, virile and powerful informs contemporary masculinity, and fatness is seen as oppositional to each of these.

The specific location of fat on our bodies may suggest particular affiliations with femininity or masculinity, with an hourglass shape being associated with female bodies. Large and hanging bellies may hide genitalia and render bodies unintelligible. Supersized bodies may generally be viewed as unsexed, with secondary sexual characteristics such as broader shoulders or breasts being less obvious. In some fat people, the location of fat can also sexualize body parts that aren't traditionally viewed as erogenous—Kotow writes about superfat women whose upper arm fat is constantly groped by admirers (2023, 70). For men, thickness may be desirable in the context of a football player's physique, but curvy flowing fat may be deemed overly feminine. Of course, there are deep contradictions in these "rules" because they are no more "real" than gender itself—rather, the shape and placement of fat may perform masculinity, femininity, androgyny or other gendered tellings in different ways dependent on context.

While the gendered messages of fat are unstable, there are nonetheless specific impacts of fat and fatphobia for people whose identity is beyond the gender binary. Because fat placement can make a body look or feel more or less masculine or feminine, fat trans and non-binary people may feel especially alienated by or celebrated by fat. The emergence of plump breasts on a trans girl newly on estrogen may be as much of a cause for joy as the blooming chest of a trans boy is a source of despair. Rounded hips and a swelling belly can help some bodies pass but can hinder other bodies from feeling authentic in their gender identity. Some of the problem here is a lack of expansiveness in our understanding of possible gender stories—there are as many ways to be in a gendered body as there are to be in any body, and no "right" or "wrong" way to any of them, but within the world of gender as performance, some performances nail it and others may require greater persuasion. It is perhaps unsurprising that there is a huge incidence of eating disorder diagnoses among trans people—weight maintenance may feel like a way to control a body that feels out of control. Among non-binary folks, the emergence of an androgynous aesthetic that is highly reliant on a lean and young physique may render rounder they/thems less visible in ways that can be deeply hurtful.

Trans-affirming medical settings may acknowledge gender identity while still maligning fat; many doctors refuse gender-affirming surgeries or other gender-affirming care to people over specific BMI cutoffs. Anecdotally, one doctor who treated trans youth admitted to a researcher that he wished he could police the weight of all young people but could only use his authority over trans young folk by withholding puberty blockers and/or hormone treatments to kids over set BMI categories.

Looking at the specific topic of gender transition raises important questions. Trans lives and trans scholarship leads with the idea that it is meaningful, if not essential, to seek a body that affirms one's internal state. Fat Studies, by contrast, suggests that the unaltered body is correct and that attempts to modify the body are dangerous and regressive. Fat Studies scholar Francis Ray White notes that "While certain strands of fat and trans discourses disagree over the malleability of the body, strangely they converge when they deploy this discourse to promote the liberatory potential of feeling 'at home' in one's body" (2014, 92). White explores the specific intersection of fat and trans identities through both literature and personal experience, notably asking:

> Perhaps what a fuller consideration of the intersection of fat and trans discourse can begin to do then, is address the question of how, or if, longing for a flat chest is any different from longing for a flat stomach.
> (2014, 93)

It is notable that mainstream culture views body modification through diet as completely normal while seeing gender transition as dramatic and radical. I would argue that we are always amending our "natural" bodies and that some degree of body management is simply part of the human experience. Asking *why* we seek specific body changes and eschew others, however, may allow for a critical reckoning of the choices that we make and the ways we plan to live (and spend our money!) going forward, especially in thinking about fat and gender.

SEXUALITY

There are distinctions and overlaps in talking about gender and sexuality. Some of the ways we think about our gendered bodies may implicate what we choose to do with those bodies in the realm of sexual activities and sexual identities. These realms are not the same, but neither are they completely independent of one another. Fat is implicated in thinking through both gender and sexuality in similar and different ways.

Fat and queer people may find that there is more room in some queer spaces for a politics of fat desirability. Identities such as "butch" and "bear" may explicitly celebrate bigger bodies as worthy of sexual attention. Without seeking to essentialize, the expectations of bodies around size, but also gender performance, may vary in queer spaces, and a more expansive view of body size is sometimes allowed. That said, there is plenty of policing of size in queer space. Gay men's spaces can be virulently fatphobic, with the expectation of sculpted and highly maintained bodies. As queer culture is increasingly pulled out of the closet, it is informed by some of the same aesthetic impulses that are at play in the broader culture; other influences such as drag aesthetics may flow from queer space into the mainstream. That said, the visual cues for queer life can sometimes uphold or even extend fat shaming narratives. Fundamentally, queer spaces are not independent of the fatphobia of all spaces, but may frame expectations through different lenses of aesthetics and desirability.

The aesthetic flexibility of some queer spaces may come from some of the ways that fat and queer activism grew alongside one another. Many of the fat activists of the civil rights movements of the 1960s drew from their experiences in gay and lesbian organizing, and there is a significant overlap among mainstream fat and queer activisms. Cooper's 2016 book *Fat Activism* explores the significant congruity and sharing of tactics and approaches between fat and queer activism, and specifically by fat, queer activists. While this congruency has been fruitful, it hasn't been entirely without controversy.

Lind considers the ways that fat activism has used queer modalities to inform fat activism, including a focus on camp, disruption and other forms of playful action (2020). That said, Lind explores the ways that these modalities can be couched in uninformed whiteness, exploring which bodies can afford to transgress in specific ways and who can afford to reclaim difference. She asks,

> What would it mean to engage in a queer anti-racist politic grounded in the politics of the body? One that takes seriously the contributions of how bodies read and are read, and also understands ideologies of race to be marking and unmarking bodies in fundamentally arbitrary ways? A thickened politics of recognition is needed, I think, to understand how whiteness operates and where it presents itself.
>
> (2020, 192)

The spectacle of fat reclamation may draw from similar impulses to the spectacle of queer camp. The glee of an anti-establishment narrative may allow for a rejection of a range of different rule systems. At the same time—there are many queer folks on diets. There are gay men in tailored suits, femmes in frothy ruffles. Queer desire does not always predict an anti-establishment orientation, nor a commitment to rejecting all of society's rules. For identities that have been diminished or reviled, access to livability may remain sporadic. For some, taking on a disruptive stance may enhance livability, allowing for a flamboyant joy in rich flesh. For others, too many shifts outside of normative status may present threats. Our adjudication of this algorithm may also shift across place and time—the fat activist T-shirt may work at the Dyke March but not in other spaces. Activism which draws from spectacle may truly affirm some folks, but may put others at significant risk.

Andre Leon Talley's memoir *The Chiffon Trenches* explores the battles of living as a Black queer man in the fashion industry. Talley overcomes a range of different challenges but his body ultimately betrays him by becoming fat, and this struggle stays with him until his death (Talley 2020). Talley's life as a significant influencer of fashion systems is informed by his experiences as a queer Black man. Yet his experience with fat is wrapped up in shame, and indeed, speaks to his inability to stay within fashion space as his size grows. He adopts a costume of a particular style of voluminous

dress, abandoning the range of garments which brought him joy
prior to his body's growth. What could have happened if Talley's
experience of fat pushed even further into fashion revolution, rather
than slinking away from fashion back into a new closet?

There is obviously no singular fat and queer story. There are
innumerable queer communities, each with their own cultures and
community mores. For fat queer folks, however, there may be
specific impacts of fatphobia regardless of the aesthetic standards of
their spaces. The cumulative impact of homophobia and fatphobia,
and the stereotypes of both as examples of excess, may make access
to employment and housing more challenging. For queer couples,
family building may often involve engagement with fertility systems that can centre anti-fat and homophobic approaches. Mainstream systems such as banking, education, government offices,
etc., may require endless coming out of closets, and the impacts of
fatphobia may exacerbate homophobic engagements. Being fat and
queer isn't better or worse than being fat and straight, but it may
be different for some queer folks, some of the time.

CHILDHOOD, PARENTING AND MOTHERHOOD

There are specific challenges that face fat parents and other challenges
faced by parents of fat kids—and of course, these conditions can often
coincide. Parents are seen as entirely responsible for their children's
development and success, with myriad other influences and impacts
ignored. Childhood obesity has become even more demonized than
obesity in adults, with fearmongering campaigns extending through
public health agencies, schools and, of course, healthcare settings.

Known factors which positively contribute to children's lifelong
health, such as access to education, clean drinking water, a variety of
foods, and safe, stable living environments, do not seem to garner
the same attention—or funding—as the campaign to (fruitlessly, thus
far) end childhood obesity. Michelle Obama centred the fight
against childhood obesity—targeting both parents and children—as
the cornerstone of her activism while First Lady of the US. Importantly, this political activism was rooted in the specific, personal fears
of a mother with growing children:

Shortly after President Obama was elected to the White House in 2008, first lady Michelle Obama divulged some sensitive personal details: The Obama children, Malia and Sasha, were gaining weight. In interviews and speeches, she described her worry about her family's health and a pediatrician's warning that her daughter's body mass index (BMI) was creeping up. "Even though I wasn't exactly sure at that time what I was supposed to do with this information about my children's BMI," the first lady said 2010, "I knew that I had to do something. I had to lead our family to a different way."

(Belluz 2016, para. 1)

There are two key problems that underpin the fight against childhood obesity, and they are the same problems that dog Fat Studies and fat activism throughout time and throughout this book. First, obesity does not seem to be preventable, especially in children. The many factors which arrange how our bodies look stubbornly resist most interventions, and the interventions which *do* work are most often extreme forms of eating distress, not "healthy living". Not all fat kids become fat adults—some reach puberty and experience a shift in metabolism. Some fat kids were never really fat to start with, just slightly higher on the mythical growth charts because of ethnicity, poverty, genetics or a range of other factors. Certainly, placing kids on diets is not predictive of long term thinness unless it successfully embeds eating distress—rather, changing children's metabolisms as they grow tends to alter those metabolisms in ways that may be predictive of higher weight in adulthood, rather than the reverse. What would the impact have been on America if Michelle Obama had simply celebrated her daughter's variable shapes and focused less on physical appearance and more on livable life? How many resources could have been deployed toward functional determinants of health and away from a futile attempt to police fat kids?

The second key myth for fat children is that fat hatred and shame can contribute to a better life. Instead, many of the health outcomes associated with childhood obesity can be better understood as stemming from the impact of living, from early childhood in some cases, with a body that is seen as "wrong". The constant attempt to change a child, by parents, but also by doctors, teachers and peers, can deeply impact children's physical and mental health.

Yet the need to change children's bodies is increasingly supported as not only effective but necessary.

Children are not robots, they are wild, dynamic and unpredictable creatures, and the logic that suggests that parents can control their children's every move sets parents up to fail and seems to have been devised by people who have never met children. It is not by accident that the lion's share of the shaming of parents of fat kids is aimed at mothers. The history of mother blame rivals only fat shame as a highlight of Western society. Mothers are responsible for all of the world's ills, but given nothing more than a card on Mother's Day in the way of control or assets to bring about change. I use the language of motherhood with some hesitation, not wanting to reify the gender binary—yet to speak of "parenting" ignores the deeply gendered dimensions of parenting labour, the ways that female identified parents are still held far more responsible for their children than male parents. For mothers of colour, this is exacerbated further: as Boero shows, racialized mothers are uniquely blamed for their children's size and scolded for their failures both as mothers and as citizens (2009).

Fat is unique in its familial factors: neither a horizontal identity such as (in many cases) queer or trans life; nor a vertical identity such as (in many cases) race: fat kids may resemble their fat parents or may be entirely the outliers in their families and there are unique challenges in either case.

For fat kids who do not have fat parents, parents may not have the tools to support their children. Further—the notion of fat as mutable may cause overwhelming scrutiny and policing of children by parents who are justifiably afraid to just let their children be. Increasingly, the popular parenting advice is to let queer and trans children, for example, live in their identities. While this parenting choice obviously faces a terrible and dangerous backlash, it is nonetheless codified in much of the human services literature and advice. By contrast, a parent who sees their fat child and supports them in growing into an empowered fat adult, is almost always seen as neglectful or ill-informed. Increasingly, children have been removed from their homes with their larger size provided as evidence of neglect (Friedman 2014). There is no evidence to show that these interventions result in the desired outcome—in fact, foster care is understood to be an "obesogenic" environment. The messaging, however, is clear—to ignore a child's weight is evidence of dangerously lax parenting and there will be consequences.

For fat parents, and especially fat mothers, the blame for fat kids may be exponentially worse. Even though fat people are more likely to make fat people—at least in families where genetic relationships are at play—there is no acknowledgement of the genetic factors in weight and size. While we marvel at families full of tall adults and children, or remark upon families who are all similarly athletic or musical, we seem to be unable to accept that weight is genetic. When children see their parents suffering as a result of their weight from their earliest age, and when that struggle may include ongoing personal battles to shift weight—a powerful message is sent that the bodies of fat children are dangerous and wrong.

Parenting is terrifying work, especially for mothers. All anyone wants is for their child to thrive and live safely into adulthood. Parents who berate and shame their children may often do so as an act of love, advised by systems that cannot conceive of a safe, happy fat life. Yet this same logic dissuaded generations of parents from accepting their children from coming out as queer or trans, flattened authenticity in favour of respectability. What would the world look like if fat children were affirmed, and parents of fat children were supported, in seeing fatness as simply another way to be?

MOVING FORWARD

This discussion cannot possible address the many different experiences of fat life and how fatphobia as well as fat joy may mutate in the permutations and intersections at which we all live. Fat life is infinitely variable; fat shame is likewise dynamic and perverse, fine-tuned to the specifics of any given life and experience. The aim of this chapter is not to suggest that there is a menu of fat phobia and that locating one's specific intersection on the list will show the "truth" of one's experience. Rather, however, this chapter has aimed to consider the ways that fat life is uniquely scrutinized in some circumstances and to consider the uneven distribution of access to fat joy and fat activism as a result.

Fat Studies as a field is more committed to contesting empiricism and resisting conclusions than tying things up with a tidy bow. The next chapter will aim to provide some inconclusive conclusions about the state of Fat Studies at present, as well as some ideas about how we may proceed to think about fat people in new and radical ways going into the future.

FURTHER READING

Lind, Emily R. M.Queering Fat Activism: A Study in Whiteness. *Thickening Fat: Fat Bodies, Intersectionality and Social Justice*, edited by May Friedman, Carla Rice and Jen Rinaldi, Routledge, 2020, pp. 183–194.

Meerai, Sonia. "Taking Up Space in the Doctor's Office: How My Racialized Fat Body Confronts Medical Discourse." *Thickening Fat: Fat Bodies, Intersectionality and Social Justice*, edited by May Friedman, Carla Rice and Jen Rinaldi, Routledge, 2020, pp. 90–96.

Mollow, Anna. "Unvictimizable: Toward a Fat Black Disability Studies." *African American Review*, vol. 50, no. 2, 2017, pp. 105–121.

Robinson, Margaret. "The Big Colonial Bones of Indigenous North America's "Obesity Epidemic." *Thickening Fat: Fat Bodies, Intersectionality and Social Justice*, edited by May Friedman, Carla Rice and Jen Rinaldi, Routledge, 2020, pp. 29–39.

Sanders, Rachel. "The Color of Fat: Racializing Obesity, Recuperating Whiteness, and Reproducing Injustice." *Politics, Groups, and Identities*, vol. 7, no. 2, 2019, pp. 287–304.

White, Francis R. "Fat/Trans: Queering the Activist Body." *Fat Studies*, vol. 3, no. 2, 2014, pp. 86–100.

WORKS CITED

Belluz, Julia. "How Michelle Obama Quietly Changed What Americans Eat." *Vox*, October 3, 2016.

Boero, Natalie. "Fat Kids, Working Moms, and the 'Epidemic of Obesity': Race, Class, and Mother Blame." *The Fat Studies Reader*, edited by Esther Rothblum and Sondra Solovay, New York University Press, 2009, pp. 113–119.

Clare, Eli. "*Digging Deep: Thinking about Privilege*." Unpublished paper, by permission. 2003.

Cooper, Charlotte. "Can a Fat Woman Call Herself Disabled?" *Disability & Society*, vol. 12, no. 1, 2007, pp. 31–42.

Cooper, Charlotte. *Fat Activism: A Radical Social Movement*, HammerOn Press, 2016.

Cvetkovich, Ann. *An Archive of Feelings: Trauma, Sexuality, and Lesbian Public Cultures*, Duke University Press, 2003.

Fikkan, Janna L., and Esther D. Rothblum. "Is Fat a Feminist Issue? Exploring the Gendered Nature of Weight Bias." *Sex Roles*, vol. 66, 2012, pp. 575–592.

Friedman, May. "Mother Blame, Fat Shame, and Moral Panic: 'Obesity'; and Child Welfare." *Fat Studies*, vol. 4, no. 1, 2014, pp. 14–27.

Herndon, April. "Disparate but Disabled: Fat Embodiment and Disability Studies." *NWSA Journal*, vol. 14, no. 3, 2002, pp. 120–137.

Harrison, Da'Shaun L. *Belly of the Beast: The Politics of Anti-Fatness as Anti-Blackness*, North Atlantic Books, 2021.

Kotow, Crystal. *The Hidden Lives of Big Beautiful Women*. Palgrave, 2023.

Lind, Emily R. M.Queering Fat Activism: A Study in Whiteness. *Thickening Fat: Fat Bodies, Intersectionality and Social Justice*, edited by May Friedman, Carla Rice and Jen Rinaldi, Routledge, 2020, pp. 183–194.

McMillan Cottom, Tressie. *Thick: And Other Essays*, New Press, 2019.

Meleo-Erwin, Zoe. "Queering the Linkages and Divergences: The Relationship Between Fatness and Disability and the Hope for a Livable World." *Queering Fat Embodiment*, edited by Cat Pausé, Jackie Wykes, and Samantha Murray, Routledge, 2014, pp. 97–114.

Mollow, Anna. "Unvictimizable: Toward a Fat Black Disability Studies." *African American Review*, vol. 50, no. 2, 2017, pp. 105–121.

Niessen, Sandra. "Fashion, Its Sacrifice Zone, and Sustainability." *Fashion Theory*, vol. 24, no. 6, 2020, pp. 859–877.

Roberts, Dorothy. "The Social Immorality of Health in the Gene Age: Race, Disability and Inequality." *Against Health: How Health Became the New Morality*, edited by Jonathan M. Metzl and Anna Kirkland, NYU Press, 2010, pp. 61–71.

Robinson, Margaret. "The Big Colonial Bones of Indigenous North America's 'Obesity Epidemic.'" *Thickening Fat: Fat Bodies, Intersectionality and Social Justice*, edited by May Friedman, Carla Rice and Jen Rinaldi, Routledge, 2020, pp. 29–39.

Sanders, Rachel. "The Color of Fat: Racializing Obesity, Recuperating Whiteness, and Reproducing Injustice." *Politics, Groups, and Identities*, vol. 7, no. 2, 2019, pp. 287–304.

Sarkar, Sucharita. "'Neither Sari nor Sorry': An Open Letter to the Indian Yummy Mummy." *Body Stories: In and out and With and Through Fat*, edited by Jill Andrew and May Friedman, Demeter Press, 2020, pp. 29–38.

Strings, Sabrina. *Fearing the Black Body: The Racial Origins of Fat Phobia*, New York University Press, 2019.

Talley, Andre Leon. *The Chiffon Trenches*, Ballantine Books, 2020.

White, Francis R. "Fat/Trans: Queering the Activist Body." *Fat Studies: An Interdisciplinary Journal of Weight and Society*, vol. 3, no. 2, 2014, pp. 86–100.

7

FAT ACTIVISMS AND FAT REVOLUTION

INTRODUCTION

Talking and writing and reading about oppression is exhausting and not terribly good for your health. It's hard to talk about the presentation of and experiences of fat people without focusing on the many forms of fat hatred which pervade our societies and culture. While one of the major preoccupations of Fat Studies is offering a deep history into the treatment of fat people, it is so much more: Fat Studies scholarship allows the resistance of fatphobia to enter the story, gives information on opportunities and connections. Fat Studies both documents the creation of community and cultivates academic and social communities in its very making. This chapter aims to conclude this book by sharing more information on what makes fat fabulous—the many different ways that fat life can be rich and wonderful, and the many different offerings from fat doers and makers that enrich everyone's life by showcasing fat pride.

This chapter is framed by the following questions:

- How can we focus on fat joy?
- What does fat activism look like in practice?
- How do we contribute to a fat friendly world?

This chapter will focus on sites of fat activism and fat joy, laying the groundwork for a practice of fat care and community. Practical examples including action and reclamation will be foregrounded. While the chapter will explore fat activism, the impacts and future directions of Fat Studies, as an academic field, will also be taken up.

DOI: 10.4324/9781003539773-7

WHAT DO WE MEAN BY FAT JOY?

A key part of Fat Studies and fat activism is in the reclamation and amplification of fat joy. We have very few models for happy fat people, so simply displaying enthusiasm and energy while being fat is revolutionary. It's tempting to prescribe this as necessary for all fat people—resist fat abjection by smiling big!—but to do so undermines the many reasons why joy may remain inaccessible. Mental health is as complex and multifactorial as fat and suggesting that optimism or enthusiasm are obligatory for any population is both sanist and unkind. That said, the alternative, which is to agree that all fat people are miserable, does no one any favours. Fat people are happy and sad, high and low, experiencing all the variety of life. Where fat people experience joy—and very specifically, where that joy may be *because of* rather than despite being fat, there is opportunity for reclamation and love.

Sometimes joy exists in the mundanity of unremarkable living. As I have explained elsewhere, fat people are automatically assumed to live pathetic and miserable existences. Ironically, being large is meant to be evidence of having a small life. With this in mind, the simple act of living *like anyone else*—educational achievements, romantic partnership, travel, adventure, stable living spaces and employment—may already be a radical rejection of the story of fat. Achieving these milestones may be even sweeter in the face of the surprise of the people around you.

A major site of fat joy comes in the connections of fat community. Many fat people are isolated as outliers and experience the unique characteristics of fat life alone. Being the only person who [insert non-normative identity here] can lead to shame. Discovering that many people need a sturdier mattress or love how their fat floats in the water or need to shop at a specific online retailer can take the sting out of these experiences, not only rendering them normal but also creating the sweetness of common ground. For many fat people there can be an experience of coming out of the fat closet (Murray 2005) in which hyper visible fat is finally acknowledged and connections are made. Being with people who are like you—in some way—is perhaps the most important antidote to fear and shame and, ideally, can create the conditions for joy.

Some fat joy is found in reconnecting with the fat body, welcoming the very site of abjection and rejection. Using art, sex, music, nature or other tools to engage with fat flesh; viewing rolls, stretch marks and dripping parts as gorgeous and desirable can be difficult at first, and not all people will find a path toward this type of self-love. That said, revelling in the flesh can be a potent site of joy and transformation. This can be true for people of all sizes: so much of our time is spent wishing for transformation, no matter what we look like. This focus on rejecting the body keeps us too preoccupied to get angry at many of the other injustices with which we live—instead, we just pinch an inch or two, or pop another pimple. Yet the endless fierce critique of the self is not innate to humans—even mirrors are a relatively recent invention in human history, to say nothing of innovations such as fillers and filters.

Where could your energy go? If you decided your body was OK as it is, what time and space would you liberate? What else would you love to do? Perhaps you are resisting joy until you're smaller or better or your skin clears up. What would it mean to pursue joyful possibilities immediately, instead of using our scant extra resources to diminish and discipline ourselves? This may feel radical and terrifying: to give in to joy is understood as indulgent, rather than loving. If we think about what we want for the people we love, however, we might see that we don't want anyone to wait for happiness or fulfillment—if they're lucky enough to have any options, we hope that our loved ones will take them and enjoy them fully. What would happen if we applied this logic to ourselves?

HOW DO WE ACTIVATE FAT?

Activism, like self-care, can sometimes be co-opted by normative systems and packaged as needing to be one specific thing: protests in the street, or petitions, or rallies. What if we thought of activism as akin to any form of resistance? Given the pervasiveness of thin normativity and fat shaming, there is no shortage of ways to resist fatphobia.

Many of these different sites of activism are discussed in detail in Charlotte Cooper's excellent book *Fat Activism: A Radical Social Movement* (2016). Cooper begins by unpacking what are seen as the obvious sites of activism: skimpy approaches to body positivity, on the one hand, or movements such as the National Association to Advance Fat Acceptance on the other; thinking through eating disorders, body image and "health". Cooper examines the limitations to traditional political activism and the ways that community building may itself be a form of activist resistance. She further looks deeply at art and making practices that result in new cultural forms.

There are engrained stories told about fat that are so deeply held that disrupting them feels like heresy. The only way to change these ways of thinking is for fat people to literally tell different stories—in media, in art, in film, in literature. Further, our actual daily living, the evidence of our multiple, complicated, messy, joyful, painful lives also serve to resist the flattening of fat existence. This does not mean that simply by virtue of being a fat person you understand the deep roots of fat hatred, or that you work to eradicate it. But even if you are a dieting fat person, a fat person who hates your own body more than anyone else does, just the fact of your existence in the face of vast resources aiming to disappear you, is itself radical and exceptional.

As with all activisms, we are stronger together. Digital media has allowed for fat connection in heretofore unexpected and exciting ways. Some of the traditional breeding grounds for fat activism—queer space, academic space—continue to foment revolution, but there is also room for connection in less obvious and expected ways—through a shared love of clothes hacking, through navigating similar health issues, through experiences of similar sexual predilections. There are ways that our fat networks are, while under attack, more robust, and more rapidly proliferating, than ever before. And while laws matter, and chairs matter, and healthcare *obviously* matters, the first step is in our growing awareness that *we* matter, that we deserve better. As we can see in other activist movements, often overcoming (or at least beginning to note) that our poor treatment is not deserved, that we did not make our own destiny, can lead to a louder voice and a stronger call for change. Perhaps the most pernicious tool in the anti-fat toolkit is the extent to which fat people ourselves have been persuaded of our unlovability and of our disgustingness. Community helps us speak back to the disgust, delight in our collective freakery and eventually demand a just world for all.

FAT HOPE, FAT JOY

There are so many examples of fat resistance that it is impossible to exhaustively document the ways that fat life is celebrated and nurtured. There are events—fat potlucks and fat swims, fat fashion shows and fat fertility circles—there is art, music, drama, literature, scholarship, joy. This section will showcase just a few examples of fat activists and examples of fat joy, but this landscape is growing and evolving and a simple google search can reveal the full amplitude of fat offerings in real time.

- *Dr. Jill Andrew* is a fat activist, academic, public intellectual and politician. Beginning 20 years ago, Jill saw the connections between racism, homophobia and fatphobia and other oppressions and sought to disrupt these ills through her writing, teaching and public speaking. Jill is the co-founder of Body Confidence Canada, which awards individuals who change the landscape of public life. In addition, Jill was elected as a member of provincial parliament in 2018 for the province of Ontario and has worked tirelessly around issues of fair pay, healthcare, social sustainability and beyond. Jill's work has expanded the scope of fat activism in its intersectionality and she is a force to be reckoned with in all aspects of her work and life.
- *Adipositivity* was a project started by artist and photographer Substantia Jones. For more than a decade Jones took pictures of fat people, often nude, in a range of settings. Many of these photos were curated into a series of calendars from 2007 to 2022. Adipositivity had a big reach and encountering these beautiful photos of bigger people, often superfat people, had a radical impact. In recent years, Jones has had a series of health setbacks and has leaned into fat community in different ways. Many of her prior images, and more information, are available at adipositivity.com.

- *BBW Bashes* are weekend long conventions for fat women and their admirers. They take place throughout the US and occasionally in Canada and include both racy opportunities such as lingerie parties and spaces for sexual curiosity and events that are mundane for non-fat people—pool parties, dances, etc. There are also workshops and sharing events. While far from perfect, for many fat people these are the first places in which their bodies are understood as normal and desirable. All of these themes (and so much more) are detailed in *The Hidden Lives of Big Beautiful Women* by Crystal Kotow, published in 2024.

- *The Body Is Not an Apology*, founded by radical superstar Sonya Renee Taylor, has grown into an online and in-person community that takes up radical body love across many different axes, including fat. Taylor's platform spans many forms of social media, spoken word poetry, a printed book (Taylor 2018) and workbook (Taylor 2021) and has connected a wide range of people around the world to the idea of body acceptance that is not just about a tame version of self-care but rather connects care for the self with care for the world and its inhabitants. Focusing on a synthesized and intersectional view of justice, Taylor's work is both inspiring and exhilarating.

- *Dr. Cat Pausé* was an essential figure in the field of Fat Studies, contributing a wealth of writing to the field and expanding Fat Studies on a global scale. Cat founded the Fat Studies New Zealand conference which runs every two years, bringing together international Fat Studies scholars. At the time of her death in 2022, Cat was working on research that considered the ways that needle length and dosing for COVID vaccines might increase risk for fatter people. In addition to her individual research, Cat was instrumental in mentoring junior fat scholars and bringing Fat Studies people together through community and scholarly connections. In addition, with Sonya Renee Taylor, Cat co-edited the *Routledge International Handbook of Fat Studies* in 2021.

- *The Belly of the Beast* by DaShaun Harrison (2021) is a beautiful book that details the connections between fatphobia and anti-Black racism. The book is intensely readable and deeply personal, making links between forms of oppression in ways that resist the additive model of intersectionality but instead acknowledge the ways that systems such as racism and capitalism work together to police specific bodies and determine who gets to live and thrive.

Beyond these specific examples, there are increasing spaces in which fat people gather—fat dances, fat swims, fat yoga, fat-specific exercise spaces. Fat people are connecting to move fatly and without the shame and scrutiny of movement in non-fat spaces. Likewise, fat clothes swaps allow fat people to exchange clothing without the shame of being the only person of a specific size. These are not perfect spaces—someone is always the biggest person at the swap and that is complicated; movement spaces do not always acknowledge mobility differences or other access needs. A truly intersectional analysis needs to acknowledge that in all collective spaces there is still endless difference. All identity based connections will marginalize some and still celebrate the centre unnecessarily. The take away for me is a commitment to harm reduction—to celebrate the burgeoning opportunities for fat folks to connect and to acknowledge that these spaces must only be the beginning, evidence that our work can begin to change the world while acknowledging that we will never be finished with the labour of demanding transformation.

Fat activism, like all activism, like all life, is in a state of constant evolution, so even as this section is written, it has become outdated. The joy of fat life is partially in its multiplicity and its changeability—fundamentally, any place that allows a way to reclaim our bodies from shame and foreground pride and connection is part of the activist project. For most people, this will be a receding goal— given the pervasiveness of fatphobia, it's understandable that our quest for pride may always be a work in progress, but the continued energy and opportunities around us are a step in the right direction.

THE NEXT PHASE OF FAT STUDIES?

This book has shown the ways that Fat Studies is a new field, a young field, and also a discipline that is still inventing itself into being. This book has explored the broad themes of Fat Studies—the specific myths that the field aims to debunk, the scholarship that documents particular fat experiences—but there is so much more to this subject as it continues to grow and evolve.

Fat Studies continues to gain traction in scholarly spaces. There are increasingly many books that fall under the umbrella of Fat Studies, some which focus on specific subsets of fat knowledge and others that focus on specific jurisdictions. As with all identity based disciplines that explore oppression, the increasing legitimacy of the field allows for greater opportunities for additional publications, which contributes back to the sense of legitimacy. In addition to the *Fat Studies* journal, the new journal *Excessive Bodies* gives Fat Studies scholars a publishing space. Fat Studies classes are still rare, but not quite as confusing or shocking as they used to be. We have seen this shift from "radical and confusing" to "established discipline" with other fields such Sexuality Studies and Disability Studies—while these fields are still controversial (and increasingly cancelled in the wake of right wing interests) they nonetheless have institutional standing. As of this writing, I do not know of any established university programs, major or minor, in Fat Studies, but it no longer feels impossible to imagine that such a program could be created in the coming years.

When I began publishing about fat in 2011, I was met with scepticism outside of explicitly fat identified spaces such as the *Fat Studies* journal. Students, colleagues, funding bodies, publications, would agree that I was saying something important, but couldn't get past my claim that fat wasn't intrinsically bad, and, sometimes after multiple rounds of revisions, would send me away. The frustration of talking about fat only to people who already agree with the central premises of Fat Studies was very irritating! Over the last 15 years, however, I have seen at least a limited openness about fat hatred taking root. I am increasingly invited to provide education in medical spaces, libraries, public health and nutrition classrooms. There is still a great deal of controversy about the claims which Fat Studies stands upon—this is a hard field to be a part of. At the same time, the total confusion which greeted my desire to talk about fat has begun to shift. Rather than fighting to write about these topics, I have many new opportunities to do so, and more excitingly, am in a position to offer those opportunities to others. Every single contribution to this emergent field allows the field to grow. Collectively, we change the "truth" about fat, contributing to a more robust, complicated and multiple view of thinking about people of size.

Of course, so much of the creation of Fat Studies is bound up in grass roots activism—the scholarship has sparked joy, but there is no question that the joy, connection, community and organizing has led to the conditions for scholarship. In common with other identity based disciplines, the lines between community and academic space are often quite blurry. There is a tension here: sometimes in the quest for legitimacy, the community roots of anti-oppression can be left behind. Grants, peer-reviewed articles, and institutional grounding skew toward the empirical and the quantitative; the quest for revolution can be muted in the attempt to get a seat at the table. Unsurprisingly, this has contributed to the ways that Fat Studies can still veer toward the normative. That said—I would argue that Fat Studies will never be deemed a field that meets the threshold for institutional legitimacy. Everything about Fat Studies—the rejection of weights and measures, the commitment to exploring feeling states and not just empirical data, the commitment to arts and other innovative forms of dissemination—they all work toward a field that will likely always be viewed with suspicion. I see this, not as a bug, but as a feature. Many Fat Studies scholars have abandoned the quest for respect and instead continue to contribute to a field that, in its radical nature, participates in the decolonizing of the academy rather than playing by its rules. This can be especially challenging for scholars in specific disciplines such as medicine and nursing where the official story of fat is deeply embedded; for some scholars in these fields there is a tension in maintaining disciplinary conventions while also exploring the new modes of inquiry offered by a Fat Studies approach.

In 2021, Dr. Cat Pausé founded the Centre for Fat Liberation and Scholarship. This scholarly group brought junior and senior fat scholars from all over the world to workshop ideas and share work. Because there is no official Fat Studies department anywhere, scholars are housed in a range of different disciplines and are often the only person doing fat work in their departments. This presents specific challenges for graduate students who cannot find people with appropriate expertise to supervise or be members of their committees. The deep contrariness to Fat Studies ideas exacerbates this issue—faculty members may not only be uninformed but explicitly opposed to many Fat Studies ideas that students wish to explore. The CFLS functions as a kind of unhoused Fat Studies department in which ideas and challenges can be shared, junior scholars can seek mentorship and senior scholars can be inspired by new ideas. While the future of the Centre is ambiguous in the face of Pausé's untimely death, it has already accomplished a great deal in establishing space for the ongoing maintenance of a Fat Studies scholarly community that transcends geography and institutional affiliations.

SO: WHERE DO WE GO FROM HERE?

This book has offered a lightning fast jaunt through the major theories, ideas and concepts of Fat Studies, as well as an overview of some of the experiences of, and stories about, fat people. Lives and experiences are dynamic—things are constantly changing and so, too, the story of fat cannot truly be trapped in any given moment of time. Fat Studies scholarship is exploding and the major themes of the field are shifting and changing constantly. This book can only begin to provide working truths about fat people and Fat Studies—an overview of where we are, ish, at the moment.

That said, this book seeks more to disrupt than conclude: to interrupt the major myths that have a chokehold on fat people and that implicate the choices of people of all sizes by arguing that fat is, and can only be, bad, ugly, lazy, dirty—dead. Fat activists talk about people at the largest sizes being referred to as "death fatties"—folks so corpulent that they are understood to be passively suicidal. Yet we all die, fat and thin. We all make choices that are associated with health, and others that are not—and we also know that these choices, "good" or "bad", do not always bear closer examination about their validity. This book asks us to make peace with death and imperfection, to take the case study of fat and apply it to a bigger logic that acknowledges that we are all only ever getting older, and that our attempts to control ourselves and our experiences are, in the end, limited.

In thinking about fat, I am able to see the connections between so many other struggles, and the disciplinary actions which are undertaken to suppress those struggles. Fundamentally, the key to both capitalism and colonialism is compliance, and fat is simply one site in which the failure to comply—whether we "can't" or "won't"— is punished. I invite us all to think about alternate futures in which imagination is more richly rewarded than obedience. I invite us to revel in our bodies as they are and as they will be, to make peace with the ways we depart from the mythologized ideal, to see the opportunities found in our variety and our mystery, and overall, to contribute to a bigger, fatter, better, richer world.

FURTHER READING

Andrew, Jill and May Friedman, editors. *Body Stories: In and out and With and Through Fat*, Demeter Press, 2020.

Taylor, Sonya Renee. *The Body Is Not an Apology: The Power of Radical Self-Love*, Berrett-Koehler Publishers, 2018.

WORKS CITED

Cooper, Charlotte. *Fat Activism: A Radical Social Movement*, HammerOn Press, 2016.

Cvetkovich, Ann. *An Archive of Feelings: Trauma, Sexuality, and Lesbian Public Cultures*, Duke University Press, 2003.

Harrison, Da'Shaun L. *Belly of the Beast: The Politics of Anti-Fatness as Anti-Blackness*, North Atlantic Books, 2021.

Jones, Substantia. "The Adipositivity Project." https://theadipositivityproject. zenfolio.com.

Kotow, Crystal. *The Hidden Lives of Big Beautiful Women*, Palgrave, 2024.

Murray, Samantha. "(Un/Be)coming Out? Rethinking Fat Politics." *Social Semiotics*, vol. 15, no. 2, 2005, pp. 153–163.

Pausé, Cat, and Sonya Renee Taylor, editors. *Routledge International Handbook of Fat Studies*, Routledge, 2021.

Taylor, Sonya Renee. *Your Body Is Not an Apology Workbook: Tools for Living Radical Self-Love*, Berrett-Koehler, 2021.

Taylor, Sonya Renee. *The Body Is Not an Apology: The Power of Radical Self-Love*, Berrett-Koehler Publishers, 2018.

INDEX